Practical Guide to Central Venous Cannulation

Rodolfo Lanocita • Massimo Lamperti
Editors

Practical Guide to Central Venous Cannulation

Springer

Editors
Rodolfo Lanocita
Department of Radiology and
Interventional Radiology
IRCCS Fondazione Istituto Nazionale
Tumori di, Milano
Milan, Italy

Massimo Lamperti
Anesthesiology Division
Cleveland Clinic Abu Dhabi
Abu Dhabi, UAE

ISBN 978-3-031-90325-0 ISBN 978-3-031-90326-7 (eBook)
https://doi.org/10.1007/978-3-031-90326-7

This Springer imprint is published by the registered company Springer Nature Switzerland AG
The registered company address is: Gewerbestrasse 11, 6330 Cham, Switzerland

Preface

Practical Guide to Central Venous Cannulation is a definitive resource for healthcare professionals seeking to master the art and science of central venous catheterization. This indispensable medical procedure plays a pivotal role in diverse clinical settings, ranging from critical care to oncology, offering essential routes for medication administration, fluid therapy, and patient monitoring.

This guide is dedicated to the dedicated professionals involved in every aspect of central venous catheterization, from the initial vein puncture to the resolution of mechanical challenges associated with central venous line malfunctions.

The book opens with a comprehensive exploration of the anatomy and physiology of the central venous system, laying a robust foundation for understanding the key structures and landmarks critical for successful catheter placement. Step-by-step procedural instructions, including the integration of ultrasound guidance, are meticulously detailed to ensure both safety and efficiency in practice.

Recognizing the importance of complications management, this guide provides an in-depth discussion of potential adverse events, emphasizing early detection and prompt intervention. Developed through the collaborative efforts of anesthesiologists, interventional radiologists, and other multidisciplinary experts, the content reflects collective expertise and clinical insight.

Designed to cater to healthcare professionals across all experience levels—from novice trainees to seasoned practitioners—this guide offers a holistic, evidence-based approach to improving patient outcomes, minimizing complications, and elevating the standard of care in diverse clinical environments.

We hope that *Practical Guide to Central Venous Cannulation* becomes an essential tool in your practice, empowering you to perform this vital procedure confidently and precisely.

Milan, Italy — Rodolfo Lanocita
Abu Dhabi, UAE — Massimo Lamperti

Acknowledgments

This book is the culmination of a journey that began with curiosity and a desire to make a difference in central vascular access. Reflecting on the years that brought me to this point, I am grateful for those who walked beside me.

To my beloved wife, Alessandra: your unwavering support, patience, and encouragement have been my anchor. You have stood by me through every challenge, cheered for every success, and believed in me even when I doubted myself. This work exists because of your love and strength.

To my incredible daughters, Giulia and Cecilia: thank you for being my inspiration and, sometimes, my courageous volunteers. Your willingness to help—whether by being models for ultrasound demonstrations during courses or simply offering your support—has meant more than I can express. You both have constantly reminded me why I strive to improve this field.

I sincerely thank my colleagues and the countless nurses who have worked alongside me. Your dedication to patient care and your research contributions have been instrumental in shaping this field. Together, we have navigated the complexities of clinical practice and forged new paths in the science of vascular access.

The world of central vascular access has undergone remarkable changes over the past two decades, driven by the collaboration of multiple specialities. Yet, we are far from achieving the universal safety and accessibility that patients deserve. This book celebrates how far we've come and is a call to action for what lies ahead.

To all who have supported me on this journey—family, friends, colleagues, and students—this work is a testament to our shared vision: a world where central vascular access is safe, effective, and universally practiced with excellence.

With heartfelt gratitude

Abu Dhabi, UAE Massimo Lamperti

Contents

Introduction

1

Rodolfo Lanocita and Alice Phillips

The Vital Role of Central Venous Cannulation in Modern Medical Practice

Main Roles of Central Venous Catheters

Access to Critical Therapies

Central venous cannulation (CVC) serves as a gateway to delivering essential therapies to patients with complex medical needs. By gaining access to the central venous system, healthcare providers can administer fluids, blood products, medications, and nutritional support with precision and efficacy. This direct route bypasses peripheral veins, enabling the rapid infusion of large volumes of fluids or potent medications, crucial in emergencies such as severe sepsis, trauma, or hemodynamic instability.

Hemodynamic Monitoring and Optimization

In addition to therapy delivery, central venous cannulation facilitates continuous hemodynamic monitoring and optimization, particularly in critically ill patients requiring intensive care. Central venous pressure (CVP) monitoring provides valuable insights into the patient's intravascular volume status, cardiac function, and response to therapy. By assessing CVP trends, healthcare providers can titrate fluid resuscitation, vasopressor support, and inotropic agents to maintain hemodynamic stability and prevent complications such as organ dysfunction or shock.

Facilitating Diagnostic and Therapeutic Procedures

Central venous access serves as a conduit for performing a myriad of diagnostic and therapeutic procedures essential for patient management. These include central venous oxygen saturation ($ScvO_2$) monitoring to guide resuscitation in septic shock, insertion of pulmonary artery catheters for advanced hemodynamic monitoring, and administration of contrast agents for imaging studies, such as computed tomography (CT), angiography, or cardiac catheterization. Moreover, central venous cannulation enables the sampling of blood for laboratory analyses, facilitating the timely assessment of electrolyte imbalances, metabolic derangements, and blood cultures to guide treatment decisions.

R. Lanocita
Department of Radiology and Interventional Radiology, IRCCS Fondazione Istituto Nazionale Tumori di, Milano, Milan, Italy
e-mail: Rodolfo.Lanocita@istitutotumori.mi.it

A. Phillips (✉)
Postgraduation School in Radiodiagnostics, Università degli Studi di Milano, Milan, Italy
e-mail: alice.phillips@unimi.it

R. Lanocita, M. Lamperti (eds.), *Practical Guide to Central Venous Cannulation*,
https://doi.org/10.1007/978-3-031-90326-7_1

Access for Dialysis or Plasmapheresis

Central venous catheters (CVCs) are crucial for dialysis and plasmapheresis/apheresis due to their ability to provide reliable, high-volume access to the bloodstream.

- Dialysis requires the rapid removal and return of large volumes of blood to filter out waste products. CVCs, typically placed in large veins like the internal jugular, subclavian, or femoral veins, facilitate this process by allowing high blood flow rates. In acute or emergency situations where dialysis is urgently needed, CVCs offer quick and immediate vascular access. This is critical for patients with acute kidney injury or those awaiting the maturation of a permanent vascular access like an arteriovenous fistula. Moreover, for patients who are not yet candidates for or are transitioning to permanent dialysis access, CVCs serve as a temporary but effective solution.
- Plasmapheresis involves removing plasma from the blood and replacing it with donor plasma or a plasma substitute. CVCs enable the efficient handling of the large volumes of plasma required for this procedure. Similar to dialysis, plasmapheresis often needs to be performed urgently in conditions like autoimmune diseases or severe infections. CVCs provide the necessary rapid and reliable venous access. The use of CVCs reduces the time needed to perform the procedure and minimizes the risk of complications associated with repeated needle insertions into peripheral veins.

Long-Term Venous Access for Oncologic Patients

CVC is particularly important for oncologic patients due to the intensive and prolonged nature of their treatment. These devices provide a stable and reliable access route for administering chemotherapy, which can be harsh on peripheral veins and requires precise delivery. It also facilitates the infusion of other medications, such as antibiotics and pain management drugs, as well as the administration of blood products and nutritional support. Additionally, CVC allows for frequent blood sampling without repeated needle sticks, reducing discomfort and the risk of infection. This comprehensive access is crucial for managing the complex and multifaceted treatment regimens typical in cancer care.

Venous Access When Peripheral Access Is Unavailable

Central venous catheterization is essential when peripheral access is unavailable as it ensures reliable and immediate access to the vascular system, especially for high-volume or high-concentration infusions that peripheral veins cannot handle. This is particularly useful in the following:

- Total parenteral nutrition (TPN): for patients unable to receive nutrition orally or enterally, TPN through a central line provides essential nutrients directly into the bloodstream.
- Large volume resuscitation: in cases of severe dehydration, blood loss, or shock, large volumes of fluids or blood products are needed rapidly. Central lines enable swift and effective infusion.

Clinical Scenarios Highlighting the Importance of Central Venous Access

Emergency and Critical Care

In emergency and critical care settings, peripheral venous access may be compromised due to shock, severe dehydration, or difficult vascular anatomy. CVCs provide a secure and immediate route for the following:

- Rapid administration of vasopressors and inotropes to support blood pressure and cardiac output
- Delivery of sedatives, anesthetics, and other critical medications
- Initiation of life-saving interventions, such as central venous extracorporeal membrane oxygenation (ECMO)

Oncology

Oncologic patients often have challenging venous access due to previous treatments, frequent blood draws, and the nature of their disease. CVCs are vital for the following:

- Long-term chemotherapy, reducing the need for multiple needle sticks and preserving peripheral veins
- Administration of supportive care medications, including antibiotics, antiemetics, and pain management drugs
- Facilitating the delivery of blood products and nutritional support

Long-Term Therapy

Patients requiring long-term intravenous therapy, such as those with chronic infections needing prolonged antibiotic courses, benefit from central venous access. CVCs allow for the following:

- Consistent and reliable delivery of antibiotics over extended periods
- Enhanced patient mobility and comfort compared to peripheral IV lines, which require frequent changes and can cause irritation

Considering all these different scenarios, physicians and interventional radiologists must be aware of the various catheters available and select these depending on the specific clinical indication and purpose of use. Here, you can find a summary list of catheters with their main characteristics and indications (Table 1.1).

Table 1.1 Type of CVCs

Category	Use	Image	Characteristics	Indications
Short-term catheter *Temporary CVC access*	Maximum 10–15 days	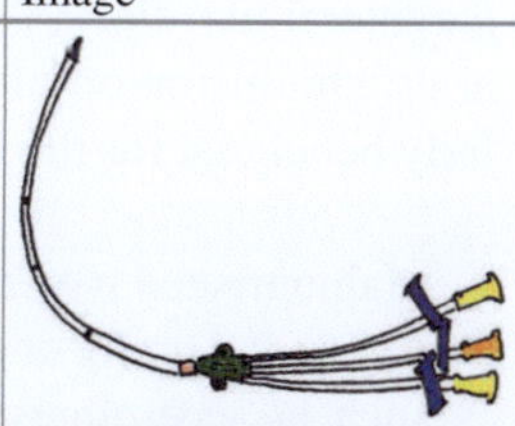	Percutaneously inserted Nontunneled Noncuffed	Acute care needs (e.g., operating theater and intensive care)
Mid-term catheter	Weeks to 3 months	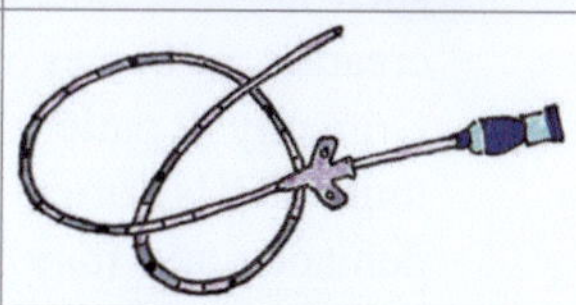	Tunneled Uncuffed	Up to 3 months for intensive antibiotic treatment
Long-term catheter (e.g., *Port-a-Cath*)	Years	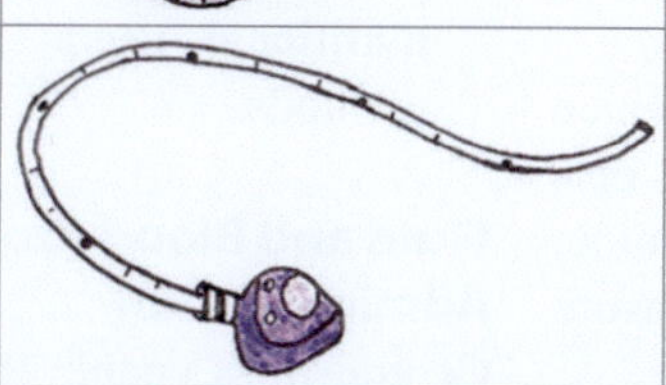	Totally implantable venous access device	Cyclical access required (oncologic patients for chemotherapy) Compatible with CT power injection

(continued)

Table 1.1 (continued)

Category	Use	Image	Characteristics	Indications
Long-term large bore catheter (e.g., *Hickman and dialysis catheter*)	Months to years	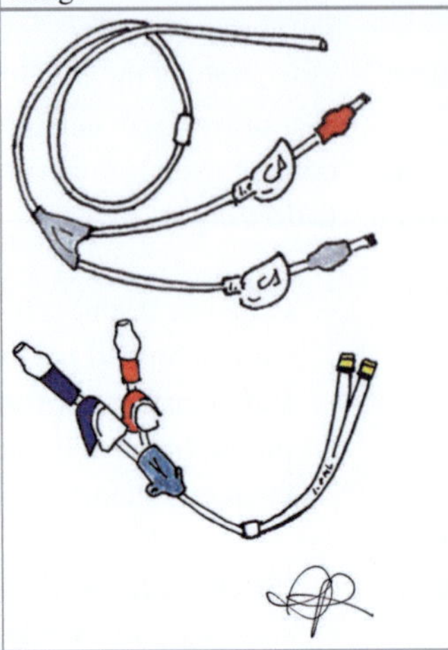	Tunneled Cuffed Single or double lumen	Specific long-term therapy (e.g., hemodialysis, plasmapheresis, apheresis, and continuous renal replacement therapy)

Risks and Benefits of Central Venous Cannulation

Central venous cannulation has become an indispensable tool in modern medical healthcare, offering numerous benefits in patient care. However, like any medical procedure, it comes with inherent risks that must be carefully considered and managed. This chapter explores the delicate balance between the risks and benefits of central venous cannulation, emphasizing the importance of informed decision-making and risk mitigation strategies.

Benefits of CVCs

Enhanced Medication Administration

One of the primary benefits of CVCs is their ability to facilitate the administration of medications that require immediate and direct delivery into the central circulation. This is particularly advantageous for the following:

- Vasoactive medications: drugs that influence blood pressure and heart function, such as epinephrine, norepinephrine, and dopamine, need to be administered centrally to ensure rapid and controlled effects.
- Chemotherapy: many chemotherapeutic agents are vesicants, meaning they can cause severe tissue damage if they infiltrate into surrounding tissues. CVCs reduce the risk of extravasation and enable the safe administration of these potent drugs.
- Antibiotics: for severe infections, high doses of antibiotics can be administered efficiently through CVCs, ensuring therapeutic levels are achieved quickly in the bloodstream.

Parenteral Nutrition

CVCs are essential for patients who require total parenteral nutrition (TPN), which is the intravenous administration of nutrients. This is particularly beneficial for the following:

- Malnourished patients: those who cannot consume food orally or enterally due to conditions such as gastrointestinal surgery, severe pancreatitis, or bowel obstruction.
- Critically ill patients: patients in intensive care units (ICUs) often have increased metabolic demands and may not be able to meet their nutritional needs through regular feeding methods.

Fluid and Blood Product Administration

Central lines enable the rapid infusion of large volumes of fluids and blood products, which is crucial in situations such as the following:

- Severe dehydration: quick rehydration is often necessary for patients with significant fluid loss due to conditions like severe diarrhea or burns.
- Hemorrhage: in cases of acute blood loss, rapid transfusion of blood and blood products can be life-saving.
- Surgery: perioperative management often requires the administration of fluids and blood products to maintain hemodynamic stability.

Hemodynamic Monitoring

CVCs play a vital role in the monitoring of a patient's hemodynamic status. They allow for the following:

- Central venous pressure (CVP) monitoring: this provides information about the patient's fluid status and cardiac function, guiding fluid therapy in critically ill patients.
- Pulmonary artery catheterization: specialized CVCs, such as Swan-Ganz catheters, can measure pulmonary artery pressures, cardiac output, and other hemodynamic parameters, offering detailed insights into the patient's cardiovascular health.

Ease of Blood Sampling

Frequent blood sampling is often necessary for critically ill patients to monitor various parameters such as blood gas, electrolytes, and metabolic status. CVCs facilitate this process by the following:

- Reducing the need for multiple venipunctures: minimizing patient discomfort and reducing the risk of peripheral vein depletion
- Ensuring reliable sampling: providing consistent and reliable access for blood draws, which is particularly useful in patients with difficult venous access

Long-Term Intravenous Therapy

For patients requiring prolonged intravenous therapy, such as those undergoing long-term chemotherapy, antibiotic therapy, or parenteral nutrition, CVCs offer a reliable and durable access route. This includes the following:

- Implantable ports: these are a type of CVC placed under the skin, providing a long-term solution with reduced risk of infection compared to external lines.
- Peripherally inserted central catheters (PICCs): these are often used for intermediate-term intravenous therapy, offering ease of placement and maintenance.

Reduced Risk of Complications with Proper Use

While CVCs come with potential risks, such as infection and thrombosis, these can be minimized with proper insertion techniques and maintenance protocols. The benefits often outweigh the risks, particularly when:

- Aseptic technique: strict adherence to aseptic technique during insertion and maintenance significantly reduces the risk of infection.
- Regular monitoring and care: regular flushing, dressing changes, and monitoring for signs of complications help ensure the longevity and safety of the catheter.

Overview. Summary of the Benefits of CVC

Rapid administration of fluids, medications, and blood products, particularly in critically ill patients requiring resuscitation

Accurate measurement of central venous pressure (CVP) for guiding fluid management and hemodynamic optimization

Facilitation of advanced hemodynamic monitoring techniques, such as central venous oxygen saturation (ScvO2) monitoring and pulmonary artery catheterization

Access to the central circulation for blood sampling, facilitating diagnostic evaluations and therapeutic interventions

High flow blood access for dialysis or plasmapheresis

Long-term access for oncological patients in need for numerous cycles of chemotherapy and sclerosing infusions

Venous access when peripheral access is unavailable

Risks Associated with CVC

CVCs are essential tools in modern medicine, but their use also comes with significant risks that must be carefully considered. Understanding these risks is crucial for healthcare professionals to mitigate potential complications and improve patient outcomes. This paragraph explores the various risks associated with CVCs, emphasizing the importance of vigilant management and preventive strategies.

Infection

Infections are one of the most serious and common risks associated with CVCs. They can lead to severe complications, including sepsis, which can be life-threatening.

- Catheter-related bloodstream infections (CRBSIs): these infections occur when bacteria or fungi enter the bloodstream via the catheter. They can result from contamination during insertion, dressing changes, or line access.
- Prevention: strict adherence to aseptic techniques during insertion and maintenance, using antimicrobial-coated catheters, and implementing evidence-based protocols for line care can significantly reduce the risk of CRBSIs.

Thrombosis

Thrombosis, or blood clot formation, is another significant risk associated with CVCs. It can lead to catheter occlusion and increase the risk of serious complications.

- Venous thromboembolism (VTE): CVCs can cause blood clots in the veins, which may dislodge and travel to the lungs, causing pulmonary embolism. This can be life-threatening if not promptly managed.
- Prevention: regular flushing of the catheter, using anticoagulants in high-risk patients, and choosing the appropriate catheter size and type can help minimize the risk of thrombosis.

Mechanical Complications

Mechanical complications during insertion or use of a CVC can lead to immediate and delayed problems.

- Pneumothorax: accidental puncture of the lung during insertion can cause air to enter the pleural space, leading to a collapsed lung. This is a medical emergency requiring prompt treatment!
- Hemothorax: injury to blood vessels during insertion can lead to bleeding into the chest cavity.
- Catheter malposition: improper placement of the catheter can result in ineffective treatment and increased risk of complications.
- Prevention: using ultrasound guidance during insertion, ensuring proper training and experience of the healthcare provider, and verifying catheter placement with imaging techniques can reduce the risk of mechanical complications.

Air Embolism

Air embolism occurs when air enters the bloodstream through the CVC, which can be fatal if it reaches the heart or lungs.

- Causes: air embolisms can occur during insertion, removal, or when the catheter is accessed for infusion or blood sampling.
- Prevention: ensuring proper technique during insertion and removal, maintaining a closed system during catheter use, and placing the patient in the Trendelenburg position (head down, legs up) during catheter manipulation can help prevent air embolisms.

Catheter Occlusion

Catheter occlusion, or blockage, can occur due to thrombus formation, precipitation of infused substances, or mechanical issues.

- Impact: occlusion can hinder the delivery of medications and fluids, necessitating catheter replacement and causing treatment delays.
- Prevention: regular flushing protocols, using proper solutions for infusion, and avoiding

incompatible medications can help maintain catheter patency.

Migration and Dislodgement

Catheter migration and dislodgement are risks that can compromise the effectiveness of the CVC and increase the risk of complications.

- Migration: the catheter can move from its original position, leading to ineffective treatment and increased risk of thrombosis or infection.
- Dislodgement: accidental pulling or movement can dislodge the catheter, requiring replacement and potentially causing damage to blood vessels or surrounding tissues.
- Prevention: securely anchoring the catheter, educating patients and caregivers on proper handling, and regularly checking the catheter's position can help prevent these issues.

Phlebitis

Phlebitis, or inflammation of the vein, can occur as a result of mechanical irritation, chemical irritation from medications, or infection.

- Symptoms: pain, redness, and swelling along the vein where the catheter is placed.
- Prevention: using the smallest catheter possible for the required therapy, rotating catheter sites when possible, and using appropriate dilution and infusion rates for medications can reduce the risk of phlebitis.

Costs and Resource Utilization

The complications associated with CVCs not only affect patient health but also have significant financial implications.

- Increased healthcare costs: managing complications such as infections, thrombosis, and mechanical issues can lead to prolonged hospital stays, additional treatments, and increased healthcare costs.
- Resource utilization: the need for specialized staff training, regular monitoring, and additional procedures to manage complications increases the demand on healthcare resources.

Overview. Summary of the Risks of CVC

Catheter-related bloodstream infections (CRBSIs), which can lead to sepsis and other serious complications

Vascular injury, including hematoma, arterial puncture, and inadvertent cannulation of adjacent structures

Thrombosis, which may result in venous occlusion, pulmonary embolism, or catheter malfunction

Pneumothorax and hemothorax, particularly with subclavian or internal jugular vein cannulation

Air embolism, especially during catheter insertion or removal

Malpositioning of the catheter tip, leading to inaccurate measurements or complications such as arrhythmias or cardiac perforation

Strategies for Mitigating Risks

To minimize the risks associated with central venous cannulation, healthcare providers should adhere to evidence-based practices and employ risk mitigation strategies such as the following:

- Utilizing real-time ultrasound guidance to improve the accuracy and safety of catheter placement
- Employing strict aseptic technique during the procedure to reduce the risk of CRBSIs
- Selecting the appropriate insertion site and catheter size based on patient factors and clinical indications
- Monitoring for signs of complications during and after the procedure, including vascular injury, pneumothorax, and catheter-related infections
- Implementing protocols for catheter care and maintenance, including regular site inspection, dressing changes, and catheter flushing to prevent thrombosis and infection

Shared Decision-Making and Informed Consent

Given the inherent risks of central venous cannulation, shared decision-making and informed consent are essential components of the patient-provider relationship. Healthcare providers should engage patients in discussions about the risks, benefits, and alternatives to central venous access, ensuring that they understand the potential complications and are empowered to make informed decisions about their care.

Conclusions

Despite its undeniable benefits, central venous cannulation poses inherent challenges and considerations for healthcare providers. These include the risk of procedural complications, such as catheter-related bloodstream infections, thrombosis, vascular injury, and pneumothorax. Additionally, patient factors, for instance, anatomical variations, coagulopathy, and hemodynamic instability, may necessitate careful patient selection, meticulous technique, and real-time ultrasound guidance to enhance procedural safety and success rates.

Continuous education, training, and adherence to evidence-based practices are essential to mitigate risks, optimize procedural success, and uphold patient safety in the pursuit of excellence in central venous cannulation. By adhering to evidence-based practices, employing risk mitigation strategies, and engaging in shared decision-making with patients, healthcare providers can optimize the safety and efficacy of central venous cannulation, ultimately improving patient outcomes and enhancing the quality of care. When used appropriately, the advantages of CVCs far outweigh the risks, making them indispensable in both acute and long-term care settings.

Anatomy of Central Veins and Factors to Consider When Selecting an Access Site

Understanding the anatomy of central veins is crucial for healthcare providers performing central venous cannulation. This chapter explores the anatomy of major central veins and factors to consider when selecting an access site for central venous access.

Anatomy of Central Veins

The three veins (Fig. 1.1—confluence of IJV and SCV on the right) most commonly chosen for central venous catheterization are the following:

- Internal jugular vein (IJV)
- Subclavian vein (SCV)
- Femoral vein (FV)

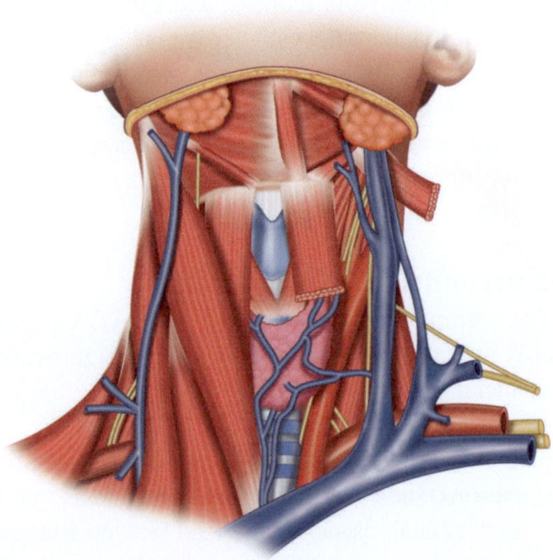

Fig. 1.1 Vessel anatomy of the neck

Internal Jugular Vein (IJV)

IJV is the major vein located in the neck, emerging from the junction of the sigmoid and inferior petrosal sinus in the jugular foramen of the skull. From there, it descends inferiorly parallel to the carotid artery and vagus nerve within the carotid sheath. From its origin, the IJV lies posteriorly to the internal carotid artery and then lateral to the common carotid artery below the bifurcation. Further inferiorly, it lies laterally and slightly anterior in regard to the artery; however, this relationship is subject to variations. The vein can be found beneath the sternocleidomastoid, omohyoid, and sternothyroid muscles at a moderate shallow depth (2–3 cm) [1]. A way of accessing IJV is usually determined using the anatomical landmark known as *Sedillot's triangle* (Fig. 1.2).

> ***Sedillot's Triangle*** is a triangular space defined by the two heads of the sternocleidomastoid muscle. Anatomically, it is divided by three borders: the posterior aspect of the sternal head of the sternocleidomastoid muscle, the anterior aspect of the clavicular head of the sternocleidomastoid muscle, and the superior border of the clavicle inferiorly.

However, landmarks have been of less interest since the introduction of the US-guided puncture technique in routine practice, which reduces the risk of complications.

Once in the thorax, the IJV joins the subclavian vein to form the brachiocephalic vein, which drains in the superior vena cava (SVC), emptying in the right atrium of the heart.

IJV Anatomic Variations

One of the reasons the IJV is frequently chosen for cannulation is its anatomic predictability. The use of ultrasound to visualize the relation of the IJV and carotid artery greatly reduces the risk of unintentional arterial puncture. However, there are documented variations to note [2]:

Advantages and Disadvantages of IJV Site

- Advantages:
  - Accessibility
  - Compressibility → effective pressure application in case of accidental arterial puncture
  - Lower risk of mechanical complications (pneumothorax or thrombosis)
  - Moderate rate of infection

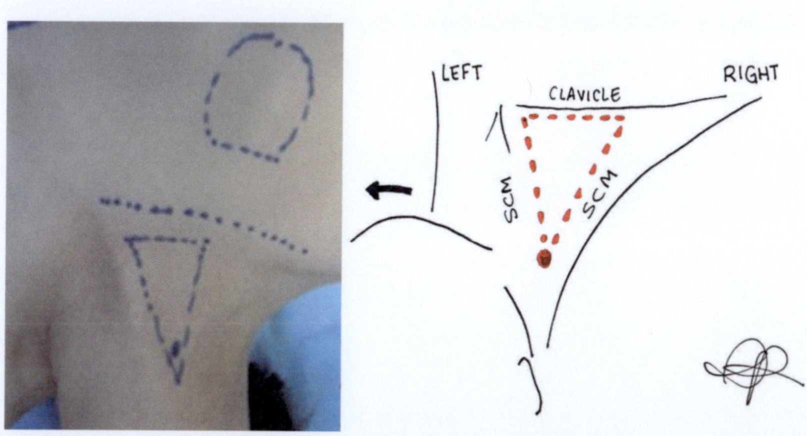

Fig. 1.2 Sedillot's triangle. Left: Trace of the neck triangle, clavicle, and socket area to guide for port catheter incision with right IJV access. Right: Close-up of Sedillot's triangle and its borders. SCM, sternocleidomastoid muscle

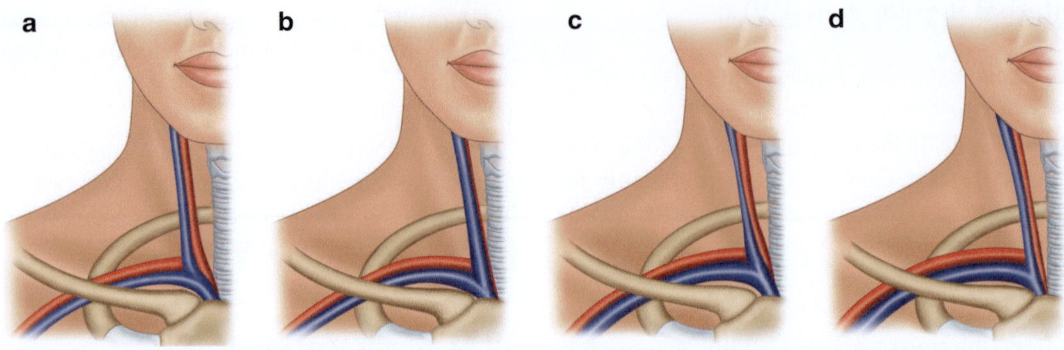

Fig. 1.3 IJV anatomic variants. (**a**) Regular anatomy (Fig. 1.3a). (**b**) The most common variation is when the IJV overlies the carotid artery, which may be seen in approximately 54% of the population (Fig. 1.3b). (**c**) Less frequently, the IJV is located deep to the common carotid artery (Fig. 1.3c). (**d**) The IJV may also be hypoplastic (13–18%), with most of the blood of the neck traveling via the external jugular vein [1] (Fig. 1.3d).

- Disadvantages:
  - Less comfortable for the patient
  - Higher risk of nosocomial infections
  - Higher risk of arterial puncture
  - Potential to increase venous resistance and cerebral edema
- Indications:
  - Short-term access (5–7 to a maximum of 15 days)
  - Acute setting
  - Emergent hemodialysis catheters
- Puncture technique principles: see Fig. 1.4

Important Tips for Access:

Right IJV is larger in diameter than the left and offers a straighter course to the SVC, making for an easier cannulation.

The right lung apex is lower than that of the left, thus lessening the risk of developing pneumothorax from accidental pleural puncture.

The relative position of carotid artery and IJV can be manipulated by a small degree of head rotation, around 10–20° away from the midline toward the contralateral side.

Avoid excessive rotations (>30°) which potentially worsen visualization of IJV reducing its diameter and distance to ICA.

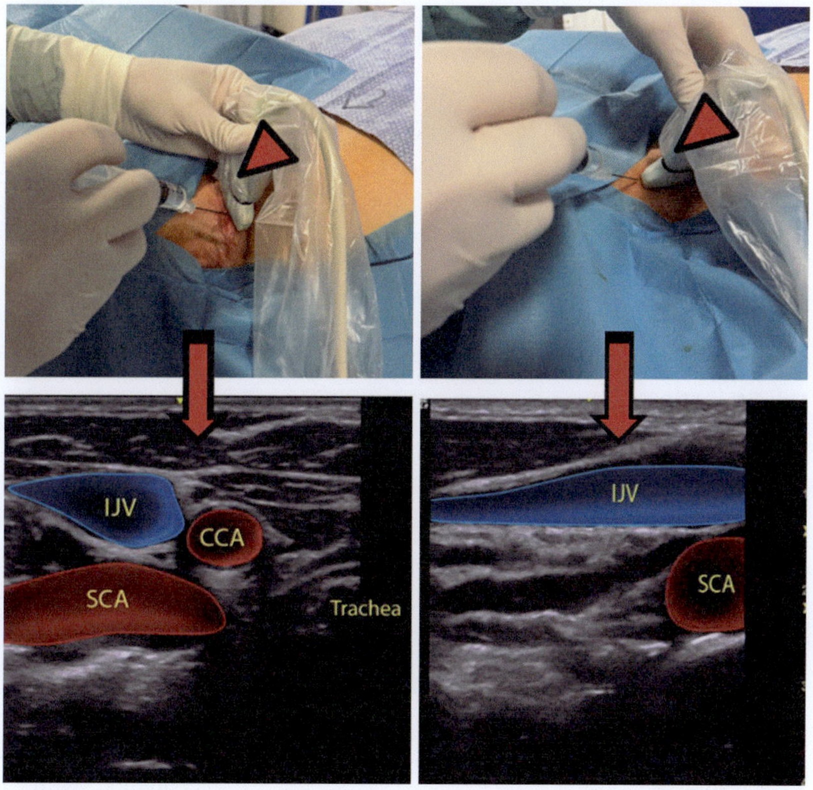

Fig. 1.4 Left: Real-time view of US-guided IJV out-of-plane puncture technique with the simultaneous screen axial view of IJV, CCA (common carotid artery), and SCA (subclavian artery). Right: Real-time view of US-guided IJV in-plane puncture technique with the longitudinal screen view of IJV and SCA

Subclavian Vein (SCV)

The axillary vein (AV) is a continuation of the basilic vein, and it begins deep in the axilla at the lateral border of the teres major muscle. It runs anteriorly, superiorly, and medially toward the gap between the clavicle and the first rib. The AV becomes the subclavian vein (SCV) as it passes over the lateral border of the first rib, until the lateral border of the anterior scalene muscle. The SCV lies beneath the clavicle and the subclavius muscles, while the subclavian artery runs posteriorly and inferiorly to its companion vein. The SCV travels inferiorly toward its junction with the IJV where it becomes the brachiocephalic vein which enters the SVC.

SCV Anatomic Variations

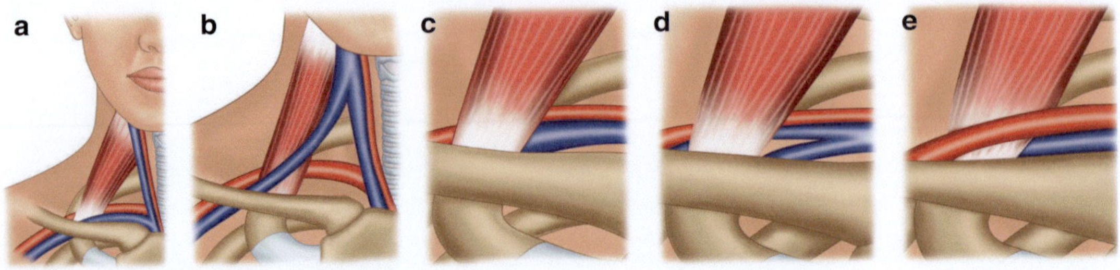

Fig. 1.5 SCV anatomic variants. (**a**) Regular anatomy (Fig. 1.5a). (**b**) SCV joins the IJV to form the brachiocephalic vein at a more superior position than the sternoclavicular joint, for example, in the neck, near the superior border of the thyroid cartilage (Fig. 1.5b). (**c**) The vein may reach up as high as the subclavian artery, passing posterior to the anterior scalene muscle of the neck. Rarely, it may run superiorly to the artery (Fig. 1.5c). (**d**) The relation of the vein, artery, and anterior scalene muscle may vary. For example, the vein may run deep to the muscle while the artery lies superficial (Fig. 1.5d). (**e**) Or the vein may split and run both anterior and posterior to the muscle (Fig. 1.5e)

Advantages and Disadvantages of SCV Site

- Advantages:
  - More direct route to the heart
  - Comfortable for the patient (+ pediatric)
  - Lowest rate of infections
  - Lower risk of thrombosis
  - Good flow rates for dialysis
  - Consistent anatomy
- Disadvantages:
  - Highest rate of pneumothorax
  - Higher risk of arterial puncture → noncompressible site and not suitable with bleeding tendency
  - Higher rates of stenosis (implication for long-term dialysis, e.g., hemodialysis catheters)
  - Technically more challenging
- Indications:
  - Longer-term access (months to years, e.g., oncologic patients)
  - Patients with high risk of infection (e.g., immunosuppressed patients)
- Puncture technique principles: see Fig. 1.6

Important Tips for Access:

Right SCV decreases the risk of pleural puncture because the cupola is lower on the right side than it is on the left.

The patient should be supine with the head turned to the opposite side of the puncture and the palm of the homolateral hand facing upward.

Needle direction should be nearly parallel to the skin, aiming toward the sternal notch.

Entering from a more lateral position may be safer in that it is farther from the subclavian artery and the pleura.

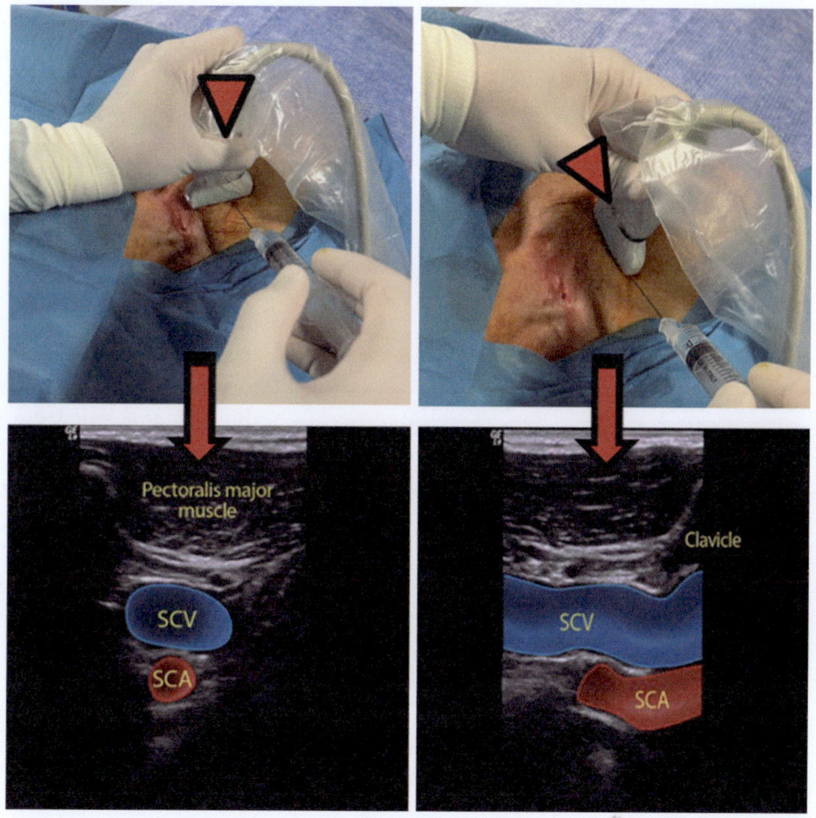

Fig. 1.6 Left: Real-time view of US-guided SCV out-of-plane puncture technique with the simultaneous screen axial view of SCV and SCA. Right: Real-time view of US-guided SCA in-plane puncture technique with the longitudinal screen view of SCV and SCA

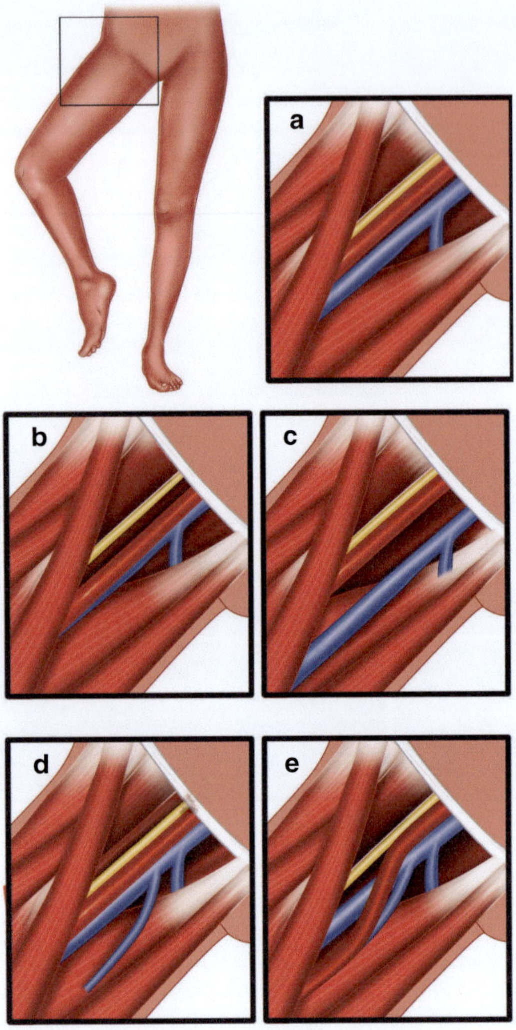

Fig. 1.7 FV anatomic variations. (**a**) Regular anatomy (NAV; see Fig. 1.7a). (**b**) The FV may be located deep and posterior to the artery with partial or complete overlap (Fig. 1.7b). (**c**) The FV may be located far medially separating it from the artery entirely (Fig. 1.7c). (**d**) The FV may be duplicated or triplicated with the location of the veins variable from the usual configuration (Fig. 1.7d). (**e**) When the vein is split, it may encircle and flank the artery on both sides in its course (Fig. 1.7e)

Femoral Vein (FV)

The FV is located in the femoral triangle, an area in the groin region bounded superiorly by the inguinal ligament, laterally by the sartorius muscle, and medially by the medial border of the adductor longus muscle. Contained within this triangle, arranged lateral to medial, are the femoral nerve, femoral artery, FV (*remember* ***NAV*** *acronym: femoral* ***N****erve,* ***A****rtery, and* ***V****ein*) along with inguinal lymph nodes and minor vessels. The femoral artery and vein are contained within the femoral sheath, a tube of fascia arising from the transversalis fascia and extending to surround and protect the vascular structures. At the inferior border of the triangle, the FV is joined by two major veins: the great saphenous medially and the profunda femoris posterolaterally. While in the adductor canal the vein is found posteriorly and slightly lateral to the femoral artery, it changes its course to become medial to the artery in the femoral triangle. It becomes the external iliac vein as it passes deep to the inguinal ligament and then joins the internal iliac vein to form the common iliac vein.

> **Remember Acronym NAV:** femoral **N**erve, **A**rtery, and **V**ein from lateral ➔ medial

Advantages and Disadvantages of FV Site

- Advantages:
  - Readily accessible site, particularly in emergent situations (CPR)
  - Lower risk of arterial puncture
  - Good compressible site
  - No risk of pneumothorax development
  - Good flow rates for dialysis
- Disadvantages:
  - Highest rate of infection and DVT (> in the long term)
  - Lowest rate of success
  - Unsuitable for measuring physiological values, such as central venous pressure or hemoglobin oxygen saturation
  - Impedes patient mobility ➔ not suitable for obese adult patients

- Contraindicate in patients with vena caval filter
- Indications:
  - Patients with limited neck mobility or upper vein thrombosis
  - Patients with significant burns or trauma to the neck and/or chest
  - Increased risk of life-threatening complications from neck access (pneumothorax, hemorrhage)
- Puncture technique principles: see Fig. 1.8 and Table 1.2

Important Tips for Access:

The femoral canal can be made more accessible by externally rotating the leg and placing a folded towel under the ipsilateral buttock to slightly extend the hip.

Place the US probe [3] on the patient just below the inguinal ligament at a distance from the inside leg that is in line with the midpoint between the pubic symphysis and the anterior superior iliac crest.

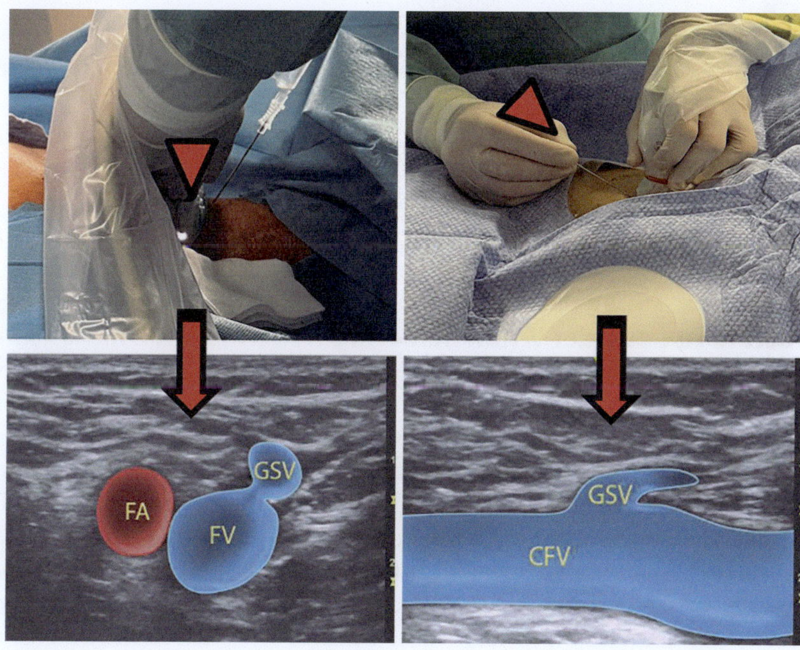

Fig. 1.8 Left: Real-time view of US-guided FV out-of-plane puncture technique with the simultaneous screen axial view of FV, FA (femoral artery), and GSV (great saphenous vein) to form the femoral-saphenous crosse (mickey mouse!). Right: Real-time view of US-guided FV in-plane puncture technique with the longitudinal screen view of FV and GSV outlet

Table 1.2 Summary of vein location selection with the respective pros and cons

Location	Advantages	Disadvantages
IJV	Most US compatible	Higher risk of infection
	Straightest path into SVC	Higher risk of arterial puncture
	Lower mechanical complications	Difficult with tracheostomy, pacer wires, or old HD catheters
	Good compressibility	
Subclavian vein	Most comfortable for the patient	Higher risk of pneumothorax
	Lower risk of infection and thrombosis	Noncompressible bleeding
		Technically challenging
		Higher rate of stenosis for HD catheters
Femoral vein	Highest success rate	Highest risk of DVT
	Least mechanical complications	Higher risk of infection
		Limits patients mobility (>obesity)
		No CVP monitoring
		CI with IVC filter

Factors to Consider When Selecting a Venous Access Site

Selecting the appropriate venous access site for central venous catheters (CVCs) is crucial for ensuring the safety, efficacy, and comfort of the patient. The choice of site affects the risk of complications, ease of insertion, and long-term functionality of the catheter. There are several key factors that healthcare providers must consider when choosing a venous access site for CVC insertion:

Patient-Specific Factors

Each patient presents unique anatomical and physiological characteristics that influence the selection of a venous access site.

- Age and size: pediatric patients and small adults may have different anatomical considerations compared to larger adults. For example, the internal jugular vein may be preferred in children due to its relatively larger size and more superficial location.
- Medical history: prior surgeries, radiation therapy, or trauma to specific areas can affect the availability and condition of veins. Patients with a history of thrombosis or vascular surgery may have limited access options.
- Comorbidities: conditions such as coagulopathies, respiratory diseases, or cardiac conditions can impact the choice of site. For instance, patients with severe chronic obstructive pulmonary disease (COPD) might benefit from avoiding the subclavian vein to prevent exacerbating their respiratory status.

Risk of Complications

Different sites carry varying risks of complications, which must be weighed against the benefits.

- Infection: skin flora bioburden varies by site, with femoral sites generally carrying a higher risk compared to subclavian or internal jugular sites. The subclavian vein is often preferred for its lower infection rate, but care must be taken to avoid pneumothorax.
- Thrombosis: the femoral vein is more prone to thrombosis due to slower blood flow in the lower extremities. The internal jugular and subclavian veins are typically preferred for long-term use to reduce this risk.
- Mechanical complications: the subclavian vein carries a higher risk of pneumothorax and hemothorax, while the internal jugular vein, particularly when accessed with ultrasound guidance, has a lower risk of these complications.

Question Which vein to choose for CVC?

- Subclavian vein: often chosen for its relative stability and lower risk of infection. However,

its proximity to the lung apex increases the risk of pneumothorax.
- Internal jugular vein: this vein is easily accessible with ultrasound guidance, which reduces the risk of complications. It is preferred for its straight path to the superior vena cava but requires careful technique to avoid carotid artery puncture.
- Femoral vein: the femoral site is usually considered for emergency situations or when upper body sites are not feasible. It has a higher infection risk and is more prone to thrombosis, making it less ideal for long-term catheterization.

Anatomical Considerations

The anatomical location and accessibility of veins influence the ease and safety of catheter placement.

Start with a vessel assessment through US scan [3]:

- *Shape* ➔ check for lumen irregularities and abnormal wall thickness
- *Size* ➔ measure vein diameter to understand suitability of catheter size
- *Path* ➔ note any tortuosity, abnormal dilation, or stenosis along the course
- *Patency* ➔ compress veins to exclude thrombosis or other structures (nerve, artery)
- *Flow* ➔ compare venous and arterial flow (use pulse wave Doppler if needed)
- *Free* ➔ from intraluminal aberrant echogenic material

> ***Remember Acronym SPF 2:*** **S**un **P**rotection **F**actor

> **Important** Always check vein compressibility! Thrombosis ➔ not compressible with probe

Clinical Indications and Duration of Use

The clinical needs of the patient and the anticipated duration of catheter use are critical considerations.

- Short-term use: for temporary needs, such as during surgery or acute illness, ease of access and rapid placement are priorities. The internal jugular or subclavian vein may be selected for their balance of accessibility and lower complication rates.
- Long-term use: for patients requiring prolonged intravenous therapy, such as chemotherapy or total parenteral nutrition, the subclavian vein may be preferred for its durability and lower infection risk, provided the risk of thrombosis and pneumothorax is managed.

Skill and Experience of the Operator

The proficiency and experience of the healthcare provider performing the catheter insertion significantly impact the choice of site and the success of the procedure.

- Training and expertise: operators with extensive experience in a particular site may achieve better outcomes and fewer complications. For instance, an experienced clinician may prefer the subclavian vein despite its risks, given their ability to minimize complications through skillful technique.
- Use of ultrasound guidance: the availability and proficiency in using ultrasound guidance can make certain sites, such as the internal jugular vein, more favorable due to the enhanced visualization and reduced risk of complications.

Patient Comfort and Mobility

The patient's comfort and mobility during and after catheter insertion are important for overall satisfaction and compliance.

- Mobility restrictions: catheters placed in the femoral vein can restrict patient mobility,

making them less suitable for patients who are ambulatory or undergoing rehabilitation. Subclavian and internal jugular sites are generally more favorable for maintaining patient mobility.
- Pain and discomfort: the pain associated with insertion and the potential discomfort from the catheter's position should be minimized. Sites that cause less discomfort and are less likely to interfere with daily activities are preferred.

Overview. Quick Checklist for Site Selection

Age and patient-specific factors
Skin flora concentration (neck vs. groin)
Diagnosis (most reliable device in terms of medication and duration)
Therapy and treatment plan (type of infusions required)
Vessel size and health
Length of time required

Patient Characteristics

The best way to tick all these aspects prior to obtaining a venous access is to keep a checklist of all the patient's characteristics, including history, examination, and investigations [4].

- History:
  - Consider comorbidities such as obesity, cervical spine injury, or previous neck surgery that may impact access site selection
  - Respiratory failure
  - Clotting disorders
  - PM, ICD, and IVC filter
  - Allergies
  - Previous venous access device
- Examination and investigations:
  - Evaluate the patient's neck mobility, coagulation status, respiratory status, and hemodynamic stability
  - Select an insertion site that is not contaminated or potentially contaminated (e.g., burned or infected skin, inguinal area, adjacent to tracheostomy, or open surgical wound)
  - Scars, PM, and ICD
  - Select an upper body insertion site when possible to minimize the risk of infection in adults
  - US or X-ray to predict depth
- Clinical indications:
  - Tailor the choice of access site to the intended purpose of central venous access (e.g., fluid resuscitation, hemodynamic monitoring, and long-term vascular access).
  - Internal jugular vein access may be preferred for hemodynamic monitoring or rapid fluid resuscitation, while subclavian or femoral vein access may be suitable for long-term central venous catheter placement.
- Procedural considerations:
  - Assess the risks and benefits of each access site, including the likelihood of complications such as pneumothorax, arterial puncture, and catheter-related infections.
  - Utilize ultrasound guidance to visualize the anatomy, assess vein patency, and guide catheter placement, particularly in high-risk patients or difficult anatomical situations.
  - Where the risk of bleeding is increased, or when difficulties with insertion are anticipated, use of experienced personnel and ultrasound guidance are essential to maximize the likelihood of an atraumatic, "first pass" procedure.

Institutional Protocols and Provider Experience

Familiarize yourself with institutional protocols and guidelines for central venous access, including preferred access sites, insertion techniques, and catheter selection. Consider the experience and proficiency of the healthcare provider performing the procedure, as well as the availability of resources such as ultrasound guidance and vascular access teams.

Conclusions

The anatomy of central veins and the selection of an appropriate access site are critical considerations in central venous cannulation. By understanding the anatomical features of major central veins and considering patient characteristics, clinical indications, procedural factors, and institutional protocols, healthcare providers can optimize the safety and efficacy of central venous access, ultimately improving patient outcomes and enhancing the quality of care.

References

1. Hoffman T, Du Plessis M, Prekupec MP, Gielecki J, Zurada A, Shane Tubbs R, et al. Ultrasound-guided central venous catheterization: a review of the relevant anatomy, technique, complications, and anatomical variations. Clin Anat. Wiley. 2017;30:237–50.
2. Le Fevre P. written and illustrated by Central Venous Catheter Insertion Guide Central Venous Catheter Insertion Guide About This Guide [Internet]. Available from: www.philippelefevre.com
3. Moureau NL. Vessel health and preservation: the right approach for vascular access. Vessel health and preservation: the right approach for vascular access. Springer; 2019. p. 1–303.
4. Bishop L, Dougherty L, Bodenham A, Mansi J, Crowe P, Kibbler C, et al. Guidelines on the insertion and management of central venous access devices in adults. Int J Lab Hematol. 2007;29:261–78.

Indications and Contraindications

2

Davide Vailati, Luigi Mori, Gianmarco Secco, and Silvia Noli

Medical Indications for Central Venous Cannulation

A central venous vessel is a large-calibre vein that allows for catheter insertion, with its distal tip reaching the superior vena cava, right atrium or inferior vena cava. These vessels are crucial for administering medications with specific chemical/physical properties harmful to smaller or peripheral veins. They are also used for advanced haemodynamic monitoring, rapid fluid administration, parenteral nutrition, renal replacement therapy, and extracorporeal oxygenation—all incompatible procedures with smaller or peripheral veins.

The central veins suitable for cannulation are the internal jugular, subclavian, axillary, brachiocephalic (or innominate), and femoral veins.

Internal jugular vein The internal jugular vein is a large blood vessel in the neck responsible for draining deoxygenated blood from the brain, face, and neck. It originates at the base of the skull in the jugular fossa of the temporal bone. It descends along the neck, initially alongside the internal carotid artery and later the common carotid artery. It terminates by joining the subclavian vein to form the brachiocephalic vein. The internal jugular vein is divided into upper, middle, and lower segments, each with specific anatomical relationships. Along its course, it receives blood from various veins, including the cerebral, facial, and lingual veins.

Subclavian vein The subclavian vein originates from the confluence of the internal jugular vein and the external subclavian vein at the base of the neck. It runs beneath the clavicle, traversing the thorax to merge with the brachiocephalic vein. The subclavian vein drains deoxygenated blood from the upper limbs, neck, and head, returning it to the heart. It plays a crucial role in systemic circulation and the lymphatic system's function, as it receives the thoracic duct, the body's main lymphatic channel, on the left side.

Axillary vein The axillary vein is the continuation of the brachial vein, originating at the lower border of the pectoralis major muscle, where the basilic vein joins it. It receives the cephalic vein near its termination. The axillary vein becomes the subclavian vein at the lateral border of the first rib.

D. Vailati (✉)
Anesthesia and ICU Melegnano Hospital – ASST Melegnano e Martesana, Milan, Italy
e-mail: davide.vailati@asst-melegnano-martesana.it

L. Mori
School of Anesthesia and ICU Cagliari University, Milan, Italy

G. Secco · S. Noli
School of Anesthesia and ICU Milan University, Milan, Italy
e-mail: gianmarco.secco@unimi.it; silvia.noli@unimi.it

R. Lanocita, M. Lamperti (eds.), *Practical Guide to Central Venous Cannulation*,
https://doi.org/10.1007/978-3-031-90326-7_2

Brachiocephalic vein The brachiocephalic vein is formed by the union of the subclavian and internal jugular veins. It extends from the sterno-clavicular joints downward, where the right and left brachiocephalic veins merge to form the superior vena cava.

Femoral vein The femoral vein is in the upper leg and carries deoxygenated blood from the leg and thigh. It originates from the popliteal vein just above the knee and ascends along the thigh to become the external iliac vein at the groin level.

The choice and preference among these vessels are at the discretion of the physician, based on the patient's clinical evaluation and therapeutic needs (Fig. 2.1).

Central Venous Catheter (CVC)

A central venous catheter (CVC) is often an essential tool for patients in critical condition, particularly those admitted to the intensive care unit (ICU). Placement of a CVC can also occur in the operating room, either before or during surgery. There are several techniques for CVC placement, with ultrasound-guided insertion now considered mandatory. However, anatomical landmark techniques may be used only when ultrasound equipment is unavailable [1]. Each insertion technique requires specialised theoretical and procedural knowledge and dedicated training [2]. This training covers the insertion process and the device's indications, selection, and management. The entire process demands a multidisciplinary approach.

Numerous devices are available for central venous access, each with various characteristics such as materials, size, number of lumens, and the ability to withstand high-pressure infusions. The choice of device depends on several factors: patient characteristics, vein anatomy, the intended use of the catheter, expected duration of use, and whether the setting is inpatient or outpatient. Therefore, gathering this information is crucial to selecting the most appropriate device for each patient. Knowing the relative and absolute contraindications of catheter placement is also important.

Additionally, understanding the most common potential complications related to CVC insertion and management is vital for preventing and addressing these issues when they arise.

Below are the technical characteristics of central vascular catheters, which are essential for choosing the correct device.

Technical Characteristics of Central Vascular Access Devices

Materials

All commercially available catheters are made from materials designed to ensure maximum biocompatibility. The most biocompatible materials are aliphatic polyurethane (PUR) and silicone.

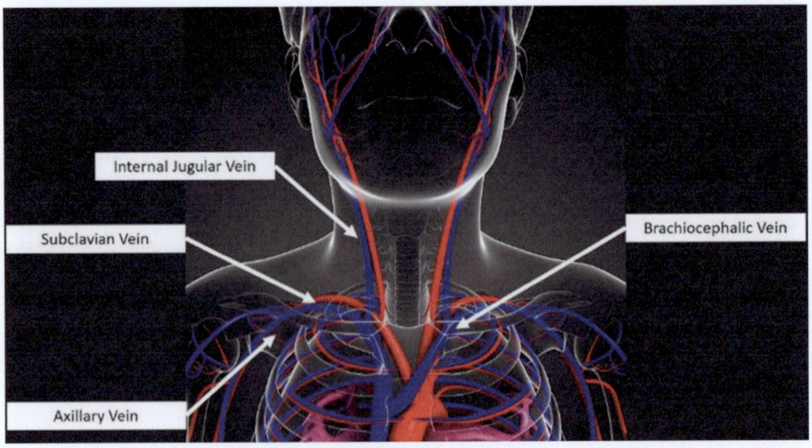

Fig. 2.1 Cervicothoracic veins

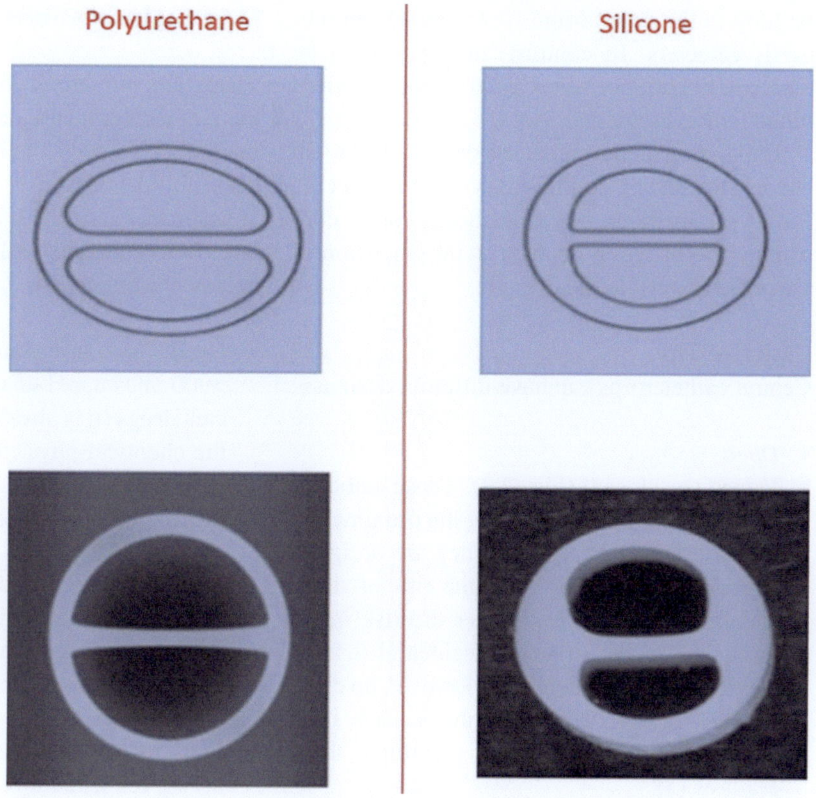

Fig. 2.2 Polyurethane versus silicone catheters

Silicone catheters typically have a slightly smaller internal diameter than the external diameter (Fig. 2.2). They are softer, have minimal interaction with medications, and exhibit lower "roughness", translating into relatively reduced bacterial adhesion.

Third-generation PUR offers several advantages, including "modulated rigidity", meaning it softens during its stay in the vessel in response to body temperature, enhancing biocompatibility and chemical neutrality.

Pressure Resistance

Silicone catheters can withstand maximum infusion pressures of 50–60 psi. In contrast, PUR catheters, particularly the "power injectable" versions, can endure pressures up to 300 psi, allowing for a flow rate of up to 5 mL/s. This capability makes them suitable for rapid fluid infusers or contrast media injectors.

Diameter and Length

The diameter of central vascular catheters is typically measured in French (Fr), representing the external diameter. Paediatric systems use catheters ranging from 2.7 to 5.5 Fr, while adult systems use catheters ranging from 6 to 9 Fr. To convert this to the metric system, note that 1 Fr equals 1/3 mm (e.g. 3 Fr = 1 mm). A critical factor in selecting the appropriate catheter size is the catheter diameter/vessel diameter ratio, which should not exceed 1/3. This ratio helps minimise the thrombotic risk associated with the presence of the catheter.

Central catheter lengths vary, and the optimal length allows for the correct positioning of the catheter tip. For central catheters inserted via the neck, chest, or upper arm (CICC and PICC), the tip should be in the lower portion of the superior vena cava, at the atrio-caval junction, or in the upper portion of the right atrium. The tip should be fully in the right atrium for silicone haemodialysis catheters. In contrast, the tip should be placed in the inferior vena cava for CVCs inserted in the femoral region.

Depending on the catheter's design, the length can be adjusted by cutting (as with some specific PICCs or Groshong or Port catheters) or by controlling the insertion depth, leaving a portion of the catheter outside the exit site.

Catheter Tip

Central catheter tips can have different designs:

- *Open*
- *Valved (or closed)* (Fig. 2.3): These catheters feature an anti-reflux valve at the proximal tip (e.g. Groshong catheters). They are designed to reduce reflux, minimise the risk of distal catheter occlusion, and lower the risk of air embolism in the event of accidental disconnection of the infusion line. However, no clinical superiority of these catheters has been conclusively demonstrated regarding these features [3].

Lumen

Central venous catheters (CVCs) have varying lumens from 1 to 7. The selection of the number of lumens should be based on the specific needs of the CVC, such as the infusion requirements of a patient in intensive care. A critical consideration is that the more lumens a catheter has, the greater the number of potential entry points for bacteria, thereby increasing the risk of infection. Consequently, lumens should be proportional to the patient's needs to minimise the infection risk [4, 5].

Medical Indications

There are numerous indications for the placement of a central vascular catheter. Depending on the patient's needs, the implanting physician and the multidisciplinary team must choose the appropriate device and the best vessel to cannulate. Below are the main indications for central access placement [6]:

- Need for infusions with an osmolarity >900 mOsm, pH <5 or >9, or irritant and vesicant drugs (it is always recommended to check the chemical-physical properties of the drugs to be infused)
- Parenteral nutrition with osmolarity >800 mOsm.
- Need for serial blood draws
- Need for intermittent infusions over the medium to long term (e.g. chemotherapy)
- Inability to obtain peripheral venous access in emergencies
- Inability to obtain stable peripheral venous access for scheduled interventions or diagnostic activities (e.g. pathological obesity and post-chemotherapy patients)
- Advanced haemodynamic monitoring
- Extracorporeal support therapy: continuous renal replacement therapy (CRRT), extracorporeal liver support, plasmapheresis, haemodialysis, and extracorporeal membrane oxygenation (ECMO)
- Need for venous interventions, including placing an inferior vena cava filter, thrombolytic therapy, transvenous cardiac pacing, and intravenous stenting

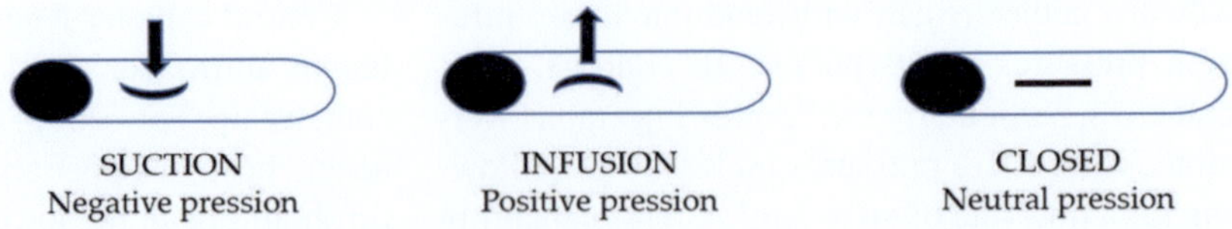

Fig. 2.3 Groshong valve

Considerations for Vessel Selection

- *Internal jugular vein*: Utilisable along most of its course in the neck, but with some disadvantages, such as the risk of infection, particularly in intensive care settings and in the presence of a tracheostomy. It is, however, a common approach for temporary and permanent dialysis catheters.
- *Brachiocephalic (or innominate) vein*: An implantation option that should be evaluated with ultrasound guidance, allowing access to a non-collapsible vein and a lower exit site in the neck region.
- *Supraclavicular subclavian vein*: In the presence of a favourable ultrasound window, this can be a helpful option in cases where it is challenging to find an exit site with intact skin (e.g. burn patients).
- *Subclavian infraclavicular vein*: It cannot be evaluated with ultrasound guidance and is thus reserved for a "blind" approach, which increases the risk of pneumothorax and haemothorax. It also presents an increased risk of pinch-off from the catheter passing through the costoclavicular ligament. However, it carries a lower risk of infection. It has a high stenosis risk as a possible site for dialysis catheter implantation.
- *Infraclavicular axillary vein*: An implantation option that should be evaluated only with ultrasound guidance, replacing traditional subclavian cannulation (landmark technique). This approach eliminates the risk of pinch-off. It has an exit site away from potential contamination by tracheobronchial secretions, reducing the infection risk. However, it carries a high stenosis risk as a possible site for dialysis catheter implantation.
- *Femoral vein*: High risk of infection, although usable in specific contexts (e.g. temporary dialysis catheter in patients with BMI <28.4 [7], polytrauma, mediastinal syndrome, emergency conditions, and anticoagulated or non-cooperative patients). For catheters placed in the femoral vein in emergencies or for reasons not included above, removal and replacement with catheters implanted in locations with a lower infection risk are recommended as soon as possible.
- *Deep veins of the upper limb*: An implantation option that should be evaluated only with ultrasound guidance. *Basilic vein (first choice)*: Usually distant from the neurovascular bundle. *Brachial veins (second choice)*: Contained within the neurovascular bundle. *Cephalic vein (third choice)*: With a 90° insertion angle into the axillary vein.

Practical Suggestions for Device Selection

Not only the catheter use influences the choice of materials and type of catheter. Below are some practical suggestions and considerations for choosing the device based on the setting (intra- or extra-hospital), the timing of use (short, medium, or long term), and the classification of the patient (oncological and critical) [8, 9].

Intra-Hospital Use

(a) Peripherally inserted central catheter (PICC) [10]
    - Primarily indicated for use in non-critical patients, it should also be considered for specific categories of critical care patients (e.g. patients undergoing respiratory weaning).
    - First-choice device in non-emergency situations, providing stable and reliable central venous access.
    - Preferred device for patients with morbid obesity when admitted for scheduled surgical or diagnostic procedures, offering reliable access in challenging anatomical contexts.
    - Indicated for central venous access with up to three lumens, balancing the need for multiple infusions while minimising the risk of infection.
    - Suitable for central infusions over the short to medium term (10 days to 4 months), making it ideal for a range of therapeutic needs within this time frame.

(b) Centrally inserted femoral catheter (CICC).
   - Contraindications to PICC placement (e.g. previous axillary lymph node dissection, osteoarticular or cutaneous alterations, chronic arm paralysis, insufficiently sized veins, and venous thrombosis in the basilic-axillary-subclavian axis)
   - Presence of chronic renal failure (stages IIIb, IV, V), particularly in patients who are candidates for haemodialysis, necessitating careful selection of venous access to preserve veins for future dialysis access
   - Requirement for extracorporeal liver support therapy, indicating the need for reliable and stable central venous access
   - Urgent or emergency venous access needs, especially in haemodynamically unstable patients (e.g. in emergency departments, operating rooms, or intensive care units), where rapid and secure access is critical
   - Indication for central venous access requiring multiple lumens to accommodate complex therapeutic regimens or simultaneous infusions

(c) Femorally inserted central catheter (FICC) [11]
   - Emergency venous access. When rapid vascular access is essential for patient stabilisation and immediate intervention
   - Short-term venous access for haemodialysis or apheresis procedures. Particularly in cases where superior caval access is already occupied by other venous devices or if future insertion of additional devices is anticipated
   - Patient with superior vena cava dysfunction due to obstruction/compression (superior vena cava syndrome), requiring alternative venous access routes due to compromised venous return
   - Non-cooperative patient with a high risk of device dislocation or removal. Indicating the need for secure and stable venous access that minimises the risk of accidental dislodgement or removal

Extra-Hospital Use

(a) Medium-term central venous access (10 days to 4 months)
   - PICC (peripherally inserted central catheter) is the first choice for medium-term central venous access.
   - Tunnelled CICC (centrally inserted central catheter) and/or FICC (femoral inserted central catheter) are preferred if a reduction in potential bacterial contamination is a priority.

(b) Long-term central venous access (>4–5 months)
   - Tunnelled cuffed catheters: Ideal for long-term access, providing secure positioning and reduced infection risk.
   - Tunnelled non-cuffed catheters with subcutaneous anchorage system: These provide stability and are suitable for long-term use.
   - Totally implantable systems (e.g. Port-a-Cath):
     – Indications:
       - Long-term use (>4 months).
       - Patients with cancer require long-term treatment.
       - Administration of specific medications, including antiblastic drugs, chemotherapeutics, and targeted anti-EGFR therapies (e.g. cetuximab and panitumumab).
       - Patients with morbid obesity (where PICC line management is challenging).
       - Frequent use (≥once a week) over an extended period.
       - Patient preference for aesthetic, social, or psychological reasons.
     – Placement considerations:
       - Typically placed as a CICC; however, it can also be placed as a FICC, especially in cases of mediastinal syndrome.
   - PICC-Port:
     – Indications:
       - Patients scheduled for chest radiotherapy
       - Planned reconstruction with a pectoral flap

- Presence of large bilateral breast prostheses
- Difficulty or impossibility of supine positioning
- Patients with radiodermatitis or other significant skin conditions
- Patients with complicated tracheostomy or large neck tumours
- Frequent use (≥once a week)

Specific Patient Considerations

(a) Oncology patients.
- Medium-term central venous access (10 days to 4 months):
  – PICC (first choice)
  – Tunnelled CICC and/or FICC
- Long-term central venous access (>4–5 months):
  – Tunnelled cuffed catheters
  – Tunnelled non-cuffed catheters (if stabilised with subcutaneous anchoring)
  – Totally implantable systems (e.g. Port-a-Cath and PICC-Port)

(b) Critical patients
- Multi-lumen CICC or FICC: Preferred for critical patients requiring multiple infusions or monitoring
- Haemodialysis CICC/FICC: For continuous venovenous haemodiafiltration (CVVHDF) or venovenous or arterio-venous extracorporeal membrane oxygenation (ECMO)
- PICC: An option for critically ill patients needing medium-term access

Absolute and Relative Contraindications to the Procedure

Contraindications for central venous catheter (CVC) placement are linked to the specific indication for the procedure, the chosen central venous site, and, most importantly, the patient's clinical condition (including underlying pathology, coagulation status, medical history, and haemodynamic status).

Absolute Contraindications

1. Active infection of the skin or soft tissues at the potential central line insertion site.
2. Anatomical distortion at the potential insertion site due to the following:
   - Implanted or permanent devices, such as haemodialysis catheters and pacemakers
   - Traumatic injuries
   - Endoluminal thrombosis

   In these cases, selecting an insertion site free from these issues is crucial while continuously monitoring for potential complications such as mechanical, thrombotic, or infectious events.
3. Lack of expertise or adequate training related to the implantation of specific devices (e.g. PICC lines and tunnelled or implanted systems) [2].
4. Lack of patient consent.

Relative Contraindications

These may be overridden by the urgency of placing the catheter to provide essential care to the patient.

1. Severe coagulation disorders (e.g. PT-INR >3.0) [12]
2. Thrombocytopenia (e.g. platelet count <20,000/μL) [12, 13]
3. Administration of anticoagulants
4. Absence of anatomical landmarks and/or sonographic markers due to congenital anomalies or trauma

For coagulation disorders and thrombocytopenia, ultrasound, combined with the characteristics of specific devices, often allows the practitioner to circumvent these issues. Additionally, it is essential to consider contraindications specific to certain devices. A helpful diagram published by Annetta et al. [14] provides guidance on the best approach based on coagulation factors, platelet count, patient needs, and the available devices.

	All peripheral VADs, non-tunnelled PICCs, and non-tunnelled FICCs (at mid-thigh)	Non-tunnelled CICCs, non-tunnelled FICCs (at the groin), tunnelled PICCs, and non-tunnelled dialysis catheters	Tunnelled CICCs-FICCs, tunnelled cuffed dialysis catheters, Port, and PICC-Port
Bleeding disorder INR >1.5 and/or aPTT ratio >1.3	No contraindications	Relative contraindications	Absolute contraindication
Platelets<150	No contraindications	Relative contraindications	Absolute contraindication
Antithrombotic treatment	Do not withhold	Aim for PT/INR <3	Maintain PT/INR in the low therapeutic range

Obviously, clinical and emergency needs will have to guide us in the event of relative contraindications.

Patient Selection and Assessment

As highlighted earlier, properly selecting a central vascular device requires a thorough patient evaluation. This evaluation must consider not only the clinical needs driving the need for the device but also the patient's medical history, psychological factors, lifestyle habits (especially relevant for oncology patients receiving outpatient treatments), and the characteristics of the patient's venous system [15]. Therefore, the following outlines the general elements to consider and the ultrasound assessment of venous access. Only by taking all these factors into account can the most appropriate central device be selected, ensuring it is placed in the best possible vessel to optimise outcomes, reduce early and late complications, and keep the patient at the centre of the care pathway.

(a) *Assessment of the patient's medical history*

Age, chronic conditions, and nutritional status. This includes evaluating chronic diseases such as diabetes mellitus, cancer, vascular disease, history of deep vein thrombosis (DVT) or pulmonary embolism (PE), recurrent urinary tract infections (UTIs), previous vascular-damaging therapies (e.g. chemotherapy), immune system status, and any prior anatomical injuries [16].

(b) *Assessment of the patient's lifestyle*

This is particularly crucial for patients requiring long-term access. Consider using devices that require minimal maintenance, especially for patients who may have difficulty accessing healthcare services. Additionally, aesthetic considerations should be considered, with the option of selecting fully implantable devices located in less visible anatomical regions (e.g. femoral Port or PICC-Port) [1].

(c) *Laboratory tests*

Laboratory evaluation includes assessing coagulation status (PT-INR, APTT values), complete blood count (haemoglobin [Hb] and platelets [PLT]), and inflammatory markers.

(d) *Assessment of vital signs*

Evaluate the patient's stability or instability based on monitoring vital signs. This allows for establishing therapeutic priorities and advanced tracking, which helps determine the optimal timing, insertion site, and type of catheter.

(e) *Ultrasound assessment*

This examination is essential for selecting the optimal vessel for device placement. Key elements of this assessment include vein diameter, proximity to sensitive anatomical structures (e.g. arteries, nerves, and pleura), vessel depth, presence of valves, vessel path, and patency (to exclude the presence of thrombi). To optimise this evaluation, a systematic exploration of the three main vascular regions (cervicothoracic, femoral, and upper limb) is recommended.

References

1. Lamperti M, Biasucci DG, Disma N, Pittiruti M, Breschan C, Vailati D, Subert M, Traškaitė V, Macas A, Estebe JP, Fuzier R, Boselli E, Hopkins P. European Society of Anaesthesiology guidelines on peri-operative use of ultrasound-guided for vascular access (PERSEUS vascular access). Eur J Anaesthesiol. 2020;37(5):344–76. https://doi.org/10.1097/EJA.0000000000001180. Erratum in: Eur J Anaesthesiol. 2020;37(7):623. https://doi.org/10.1097/EJA.0000000000001257. PMID: 32265391.
2. Moureau N, Lamperti M, Kelly LJ, Dawson R, Elbarbary M, van Boxtel AJ, Pittiruti M. Evidence-based consensus on the insertion of central venous access devices: definition of minimal requirements for training. Br J Anaesth. 2013;110(3):347–56. https://doi.org/10.1093/bja/aes499. Epub 2013 Jan 29. PMID: 23361124.
3. Pittiruti M, Emoli A, Porta P, Marche B, DeAngelis R, Scoppettuolo G. A prospective, randomized comparison of three different types of valved and non-valved peripherally inserted central catheters. J Vasc Access. 2014;15(6):519–23. https://doi.org/10.5301/jva.5000280. Epub 2014 Aug 27. PMID: 25198813.
4. Dellinger RP, Rhodes A, Evans L, Alhazzani W, Beale R, Jaeschke R, Machado FR, Masur H, Osborn T, Parker MM, Schorr C, Townsend SR, Levy MM. Surviving sepsis campaign. Crit Care Med. 2023;51(4):431–44. https://doi.org/10.1097/CCM.0000000000005804. Epub 2023 Mar 18. PMID: 36928012.
5. Buetti N, Marschall J, Drees M, Fakih MG, Hadaway L, Maragakis LL, Monsees E, Novosad S, O'Grady NP, Rupp ME, Wolf J, Yokoe D, Mermel LA. Strategies to prevent central line-associated bloodstream infections in acute-care hospitals: 2022 update. Infect Control Hosp Epidemiol. 2022;43(5):553–69. https://doi.org/10.1017/ice.2022.87. Epub 2022 Apr 19. PMID: 35437133; PMCID: PMC9096710.
6. Pinelli F, Pittiruti M, Annetta MG, Barbani F, Bertoglio S, Biasucci DG, Bolis D, Brescia F, Capozzoli G, D'Arrigo S, Deganello E, Elli S, Fabiani A, Fabiani F, Gidaro A, Giustivi D, Iacobone E, La Greca A, Longo F, Lucchini A, Marche B, Romagnoli S, Scoppettuolo G, Selmi V, Vailati D, Villa G, Pepe G. A GAVeCeLT consensus on the indication, insertion, and management of central venous access devices in the critically ill. J Vasc Access. 2024 Aug;3:11297298241262932. https://doi.org/10.1177/11297298241262932. Epub ahead of print. PMID: 39097780.
7. Parienti JJ, Thirion M, Mègarbane B, et al. Femoral vs jugular venous catheterization and risk of nosocomial events in adults requiring acute renal replacement therapy. A randomized controlled trial. JAMA. 2008;299:2413–22.
8. Expert Panel on Interventional Radiology, Massouh A, Kwan SW, Fidelman N, Higgins M, Abujudeh H, Charalel RA, Guimaraes MS, Gupta A, Lam A, Majdalany BS, Patel PJ, Stadtlander KS, Stillwell T, EYL T, Tong RT, Kapoor BS. ACR Appropriateness Criteria® central venous access device and site selection. J Am Coll Radiol. 2023;20(5S):S3–S19. https://doi.org/10.1016/j.jacr.2023.02.021. PMID: 37236750.
9. Nickel B, Gorski L, Kleidon T, Kyes A, DeVries M, Keogh S, Meyer B, Sarver MJ, Crickman R, Ong J, Clare S, Hagle ME. Infusion therapy standards of practice, 9th Edition. J Infus Nurs. 2024;47(1S Suppl 1):S1–S285. https://doi.org/10.1097/NAN.0000000000000532. PMID: 38211609.
10. Chopra V, Flanders SA, Saint S, Woller SC, O'Grady NP, Safdar N, Trerotola SO, Saran R, Moureau N, Wiseman S, Pittiruti M, Akl EA, Lee AY, Courey A, Swaminathan L, LeDonne J, Becker C, Krein SL, Bernstein SJ, Michigan Appropriateness Guide for Intravenous Catheters (MAGIC) Panel. The Michigan Appropriateness Guide for Intravenous Catheters (MAGIC): results from a multispecialty panel using the RAND/UCLA appropriateness method. Ann Intern Med. 2015;163(6 Suppl):S1–40. https://doi.org/10.7326/M15-0744. PMID: 26369828.
11. Raad I, Narro J, Khan A, Tarrand J, Vartivarian S, Bodey GP. Serious complications of vascular catheter-related Staphylococcus aureus bacteremia in cancer patients. Eur J Clin Microbiol Infect Dis. 1992;11(8):675–82. https://doi.org/10.1007/BF01989970. PMID: 1425725.
12. Bishop L, Dougherty L, Bodenham A, Mansi J, Crowe P, Kibbler C, Shannon M, Treleaven J. Guidelines on the insertion and management of central venous access devices in adults. Int J Lab Hematol. 2007;29(4):261–78. https://doi.org/10.1111/j.1751-553X.2007.00931.x. PMID: 17617077.
13. Kaufman RM, Djulbegovic B, Gernsheimer T, Kleinman S, Tinmouth AT, Capocelli KE, Cipolle MD, Cohn CS, Fung MK, Grossman BJ, Mintz PD, O'Malley BA, Sesok-Pizzini DA, Shander A, Stack GE, Webert KE, Weinstein R, Welch BG, Whitman GJ, Wong EC, Tobian AA, AABB. Platelet transfusion: a clinical practice guideline from the AABB. Ann Intern Med. 2015;162(3):205–13. https://doi.org/10.7326/M14-1589. PMID: 25383671.
14. Annetta MG, Bertoglio S, Biffi R, Brescia F, Giarretta I, Greca A, Panocchia N, Passaro G, Perna F, Pinelli F, Pittiruti M, Prisco D, Sanna T, Scoppettuolo G. Management of antithrombotic treatment and

bleeding disorders in patients requiring venous access devices: a systematic review and a GAVeCeLT consensus statement. J Vasc Access. 2022;23(4):660–71. https://doi.org/10.1177/11297298211072407. Epub 2022 May 9. PMID: 35533088.
15. Gorski LA, Hadaway L, Hagle ME, Broadhurst D, Clare S, Kleidon T, Meyer BM, Nickel B, Rowley S, Sharpe E, Alexander M. Infusion therapy standards of practice, 8th Edition. J Infus Nurs. 2021;44(1S Suppl 1):S1–S224. https://doi.org/10.1097/NAN.0000000000000396. PMID: 33394637.
16. Mandalà M, Falanga A, Roila F, On behalf of the ESMO Guidelines Working Group. Management of venous thromboembolism (VTE) in cancer patients: ESMO Clinical Practice Guidelines. Ann Oncol. 2011;22(Supplement 6):vi85–92.

Equipment and Preparation for Central Venous Cannulation

3

Alice Phillips and Gaetano Valerio Davide Amato

Understanding the Anatomy

Before delving into the equipment required for central venous cannulation, it is imperative to have a thorough understanding of the anatomy involved (see Chap. 1). The internal jugular, subclavian, and femoral veins are the primary sites for central venous access due to their large size, accessibility, and proximity to major vessels. Each site has its advantages and considerations, and healthcare providers must select the appropriate site based on patient characteristics and clinical indications.

Essential Equipment

Ultrasound (US) Machine

- Optimal imaging is achieved using a linear probe with high-frequency range (>5 MHz), which is indispensable for real-time visualization of the anatomy and guidance during venous cannulation.
- Provides accurate identification of the target vein, adjacent structures, and potential complications such as arterial puncture or pneumothorax.
- Doppler capabilities aid in confirming venous pulsatility and distinguishing veins from arteries (Fig. 3.1).

Generally, five settings need adjustment (Fig. 3.2):

> **Acronym:**
> **BART**—*Blue Away; Red Towards* ➔ it is conventional to represent movement away from the probe as blue and movement toward the probe as red.

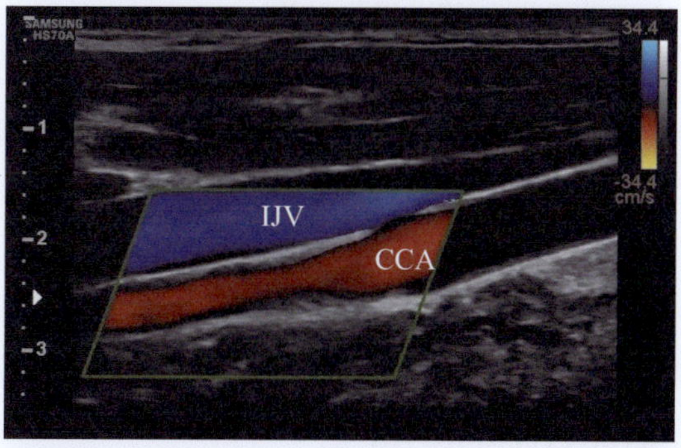

Fig. 3.1 Longitudinal view of neck vessels with Doppler-US. IJV, internal jugular vein; CCA, common carotid artery

A. Phillips (✉) · G. V. D. Amato
Postgraduation School in Radiodiagnostics, Università degli Studi di Milano, Milan, Italy
e-mail: alice.phillips@unimi.it; Gaetano.amato@unimi.it

R. Lanocita, M. Lamperti (eds.), *Practical Guide to Central Venous Cannulation*,
https://doi.org/10.1007/978-3-031-90326-7_3

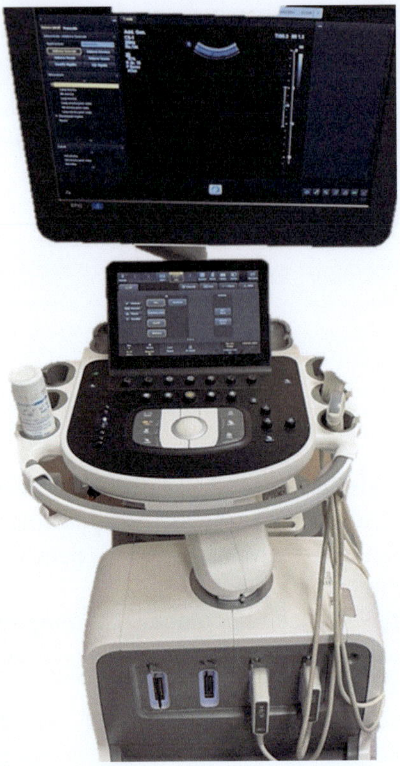

Fig. 3.2 US machine

1. *Power*: on/off button.
2. *Gain*: controls the amplification of the signal.
3. *Depth*: adjust to the minimum depth necessary to visualize all relevant structures, ensuring maximum frequency and resolution. The image is marked with centimeter and half-centimeter depth indicators.
4. *Doppler* (often labeled as color): assists in identifying venous thrombosis and differentiating veins from arteries. It is useful during the initial planning ultrasound but typically not needed during cannulation.
5. *Focus*: enhances the resolution of a determined level of the image. It is useful to better visualize the vessel wall and the needle tip.

Sterile Procedure Kit

- Sterile gloves, drapes, gowns, and masks to maintain aseptic technique during the procedure, reducing the risk of infection.
- Components may vary based on institutional protocols but typically include chlorhexidine or iodine-based antiseptics for skin preparation.

Central Venous Catheter (CVC)

- Select the appropriate size and type of CVC based on patient factors such as vein size, anticipated duration of use, and intended purpose (e.g., administration of fluids, medications, or hemodynamic monitoring).
- CVCs may be single, double, or triple lumen, with varying lengths and diameters to accommodate different clinical scenarios (Figs. 3.3 and 3.4).

Guidewire and Dilators

- Facilitate the advancement of the catheter into the vein by providing a pathway through the soft tissues.
- Guidewires come in various lengths and configurations, including J-tip and straight-tip designs, to suit different insertion techniques and patient anatomies.
- Dilators assist in gradual vessel dilation to minimize trauma and enhance catheter insertion.

Suture Kit

- Sutures, needles, and adhesive strips for securing the catheter in place once inserted.
- Suturing techniques may vary, with options for simple interrupted, subcuticular, or purse-string sutures depending on clinical preference and patient factors.

Dressing and Securement Devices

- Transparent dressings and securement devices help maintain catheter integrity and reduce the risk of dislodgement or infection.
- Options include transparent film dressings, sutureless securement devices, and adhesive anchors tailored to CVC size and site.

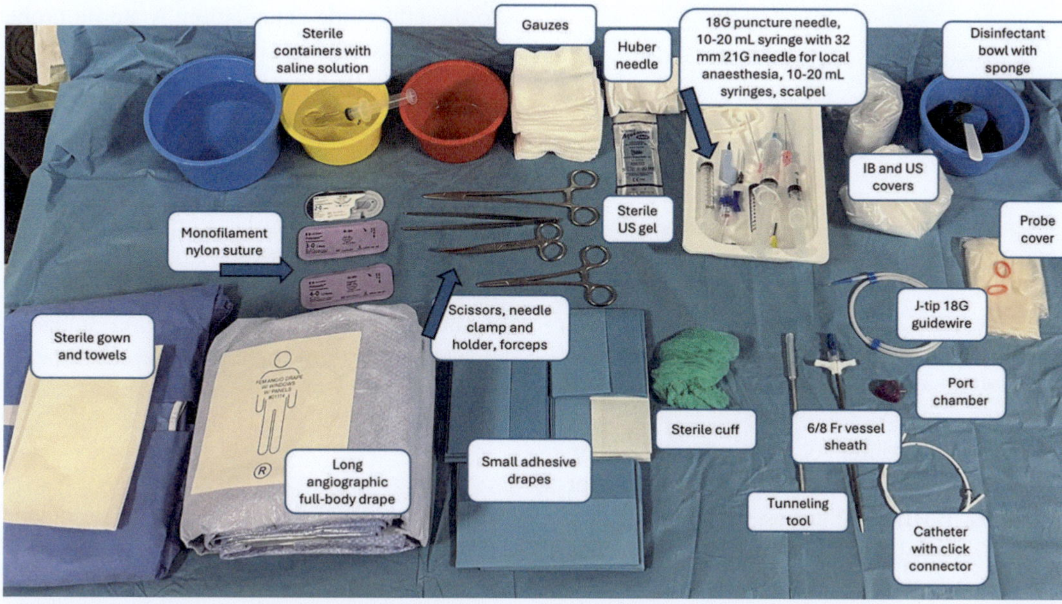

Fig. 3.3 Example of sterile operating table for port catheter insertion

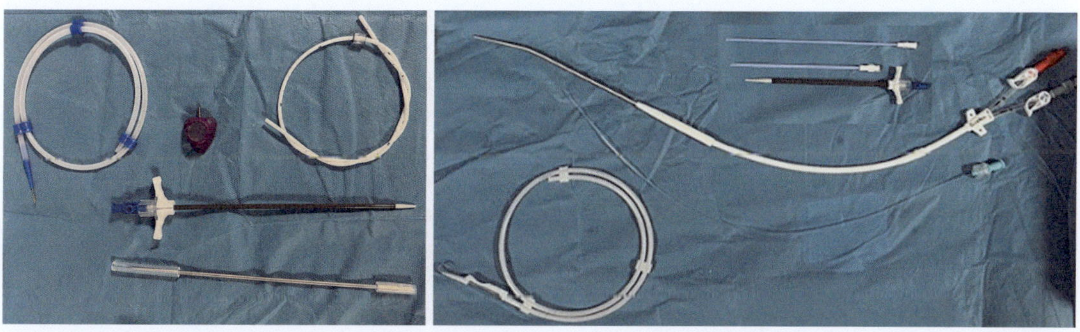

Fig. 3.4 Close up of port cath (left) and dialysis single-lumen catheter (right) insertion kit

Conclusions

Central venous cannulation is a vital skill in modern medicine, allowing for the safe and efficient delivery of essential therapies and monitoring in critically ill patients. The availability of the essential equipment outlined in this chapter is paramount for healthcare providers to perform this procedure with precision, minimizing complications and optimizing patient outcomes. Continuous education, training, and adherence to best practices are essential to ensure proficiency and competency in central venous access.

Preparation of the Patient and Procedure Room

Preparation of the patient and the procedure room for the insertion of a central venous catheter (CVC) is critical to ensure patient safety and procedural success. A checklist (Fig. 3.5) sets out a template of critical steps to be included prior to intervention.

Checklist

- *Interview*: collect all possible information including full name, date of birth, gender,

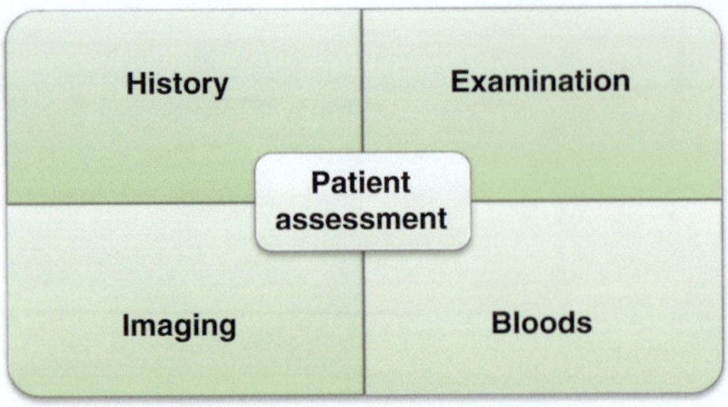

Fig. 3.5 Patient assessment: provide a checklist to target all aspects regarding patient's history, examination, recent imaging, and bloods

planned procedure, location of patient (e.g., ward or admission lounge), significant comorbidities, BMI, or allergies. In addition, thorough medical history evaluation is needed, including nature of disease, current medications, previous radiotherapy, trauma, or venous access.

- *Examination*: assess the ability to lie flat, scars or burns (surgical or vascular procedures), PM/ICD, level of cooperation, confusion, and skin infection/inflammation.
- *Investigations*: coagulation status should be assessed to minimize bleeding risks (platelet count, clotting parameters); a recent CT/chest X-ray could be useful to detect possible obstacles in vein cannulation or to support side selection. Always have a preliminary US check to assess vein patency.
- *Informed consent*: informed consent must be obtained, explaining the procedure, risks, and benefits.
- *Patient preparation*: the patient should be positioned comfortably, typically in a supine position, and the intended insertion site should be cleaned and shaved.
- *Ultrasound*: scouting ultrasound examination should be performed prior to the procedure to help select the most appropriate site, identify the anatomy, and establish the optimal patient position for the procedure. Ultrasound imaging should be used again during the procedure to directly guide cannulation. A sterile probe cover and sterile gel is required for the intra-procedural ultrasound.

Important!
Position US machine in your line of view so you can glance effortlessly from US to insertion site. The less head movement you require to switch between looking at the needle and the ultrasound screen, the better!

- *Planning*: select the most appropriate device for the treatment ordered that suits the anatomy of the patient.
- *Monitoring*: monitoring equipment, such as a cardiac monitor (ECG, CF) and pulse oximeter (spO2), should be available to continuously observe the patient's vital signs. A peripheral venous access is always obtained before starting the procedure. Antibiotic prophylaxis is not mandatory, and it depends on the internal standard practice protocol.
- *Cushion, face mask, and hair cap*: it is important to ensure that the patient is in a position of comfort, and necessary analgesia is given if needed prior to the procedure.
- *Trolly setup*: this is usually prepared during or before the patient's preparation. The procedure room must be prepared to maintain sterility and equipped with all necessary supplies, including sterile gloves, gowns, masks, drapes, and CVC insertion kits.

Important!
All team members must adhere to strict aseptic techniques to reduce the risk of infection.

Sterilization and Aseptic Technique

Central venous catheterization is a crucial procedure for patients requiring long-term intravenous access, particularly in intensive care units, oncology, and other critical care settings. The implementation of strict sterilization and aseptic techniques is vital to minimize the risk of catheter-related bloodstream infections (CRBSIs). A sterile field is defined as a surface designated for placing sterile equipment, ensuring that it remains free from microorganisms [1]. During CVC placement procedures, ensuring a sterile environment and employing aseptic techniques is of utmost importance to prevent infections and complications. The practice of sterilization is therefore a cornerstone of surgical procedures, aiming to minimize microbial presence as much as possible and prioritize patient protection from infection. This chapter delves into the principles and practices of sterilization and aseptic technique for the safe insertion, maintenance, and care of central venous catheters.

Principles of Sterilization and Aseptic Technique

Objective of surgical hand antisepsis is to minimize the transient and resident flora since skin can never be rendered completely sterile. It is therefore crucial to differentiate sterilization from aseptic techniques.

Definition *Sterilization* refers to the process of eliminating all forms of microbial life, including bacteria, viruses, fungi, and spores from surfaces, instruments, and fluids.

Definition *Aseptic technique* involves a collection of practices and actions designed to prevent contamination by pathogens and maintain sterility while undergoing invasive clinical interventions, including insertion and maintenance of indwelling medical devices.

Sterilization and aseptic technique are crucial in minimizing the risk of infection during CVC, since the introduction of a catheter into a central vein creates a direct pathway for microorganisms to enter the bloodstream, potentially leading to severe infections such as CRBSIs and sepsis.

Key Principles

- Hand hygiene: effective hand hygiene is the single most important measure to prevent infection. Use an alcohol-based hand sanitizer or wash hands with soap and water before and after any procedure.
- Personal protective equipment (PPE): use of sterile gloves, gowns, masks, and caps to create a barrier against infection.
- Sterile field: establishing and maintaining a sterile field using sterile drapes and ensuring all equipment within this field remains sterile.
- Antiseptic skin preparation: thorough cleaning of the skin at the insertion site with an appropriate antiseptic solution.
- Sterile equipment: using sterilized instruments and ensuring all consumables are sterile before use.

Aim of Sterilization and Aseptic Techniques

- Patient safety: proper sterilization and aseptic technique are essential to protect patients from infections that can prolong hospital stays, increase healthcare costs, and lead to severe morbidity and mortality.
- Procedure efficacy: ensuring a sterile environment helps maintain the integrity and functionality of the catheter, reducing the likelihood of complications that could necessitate catheter removal and replacement.

Important!
Always review and follow your hospital policy regarding this specific skill ➔ provide a checklist to clinicians to ensure adherence to aseptic techniques.

Hand Scrubbing, Gowning, and Gloving

The preliminary sterilization takes place on the back table before heading to the surgical site and the patient. A mayo stand next to the field is discretionary to the operator preference and procedure complexity.

Equipment

The following equipment is required to guarantee a deep sterilization of hands and forearms before heading to the operating area:

- Sink/automatic sink
- Sterile scrub brush with nail pick
- Antiseptic soap
- Sterile cloth towels
- Sterile gowns and gloves
- Nonsterile cap/hat/bonnet and masks

Since skin cannot be sterilized, surgical hand scrub is mandatory, despite the use of sterile surgical gloves. A surgical hand scrub is an antiseptic surgical scrub or rub that is performed prior to donning surgical attire and lasts 2–5 min, depending on product used and hospital policy [1]. It is demonstrated that after surgery, micropuncture is present in sterile gloves allowing water and body fluids to penetrate the glove causing bacterial hand contamination. Several reports are described in literature where patients' infections were directly correlated to surgeons' skin bacterial flora.

WHO Guidelines on Hand Hygiene in Health Care [2] accurately describe a step-by-step process of the correct procedure for hand hygiene and surgical scrub. Regardless of which guideline is followed, handwashing compliance is essential for the prevention of infections during the insertion and manipulation of any vascular access device. Before undergoing surgical hand hygiene, there are some key steps and rules to follow:

- Keep nails short, clean, and healthy
- Do not wear artificial nails or nail polish
- Remove all hand and arm jewelry (rings, bracelets, wrist watches)
- Don a nonsterile cap, protective eyewear, and surgical mask to cover your mouth/nose
- Wash hands with a nonmedicated soap or alcohol-based formulation if visibly dirty or soiled (total duration 40–60 s) (Fig. 3.6).

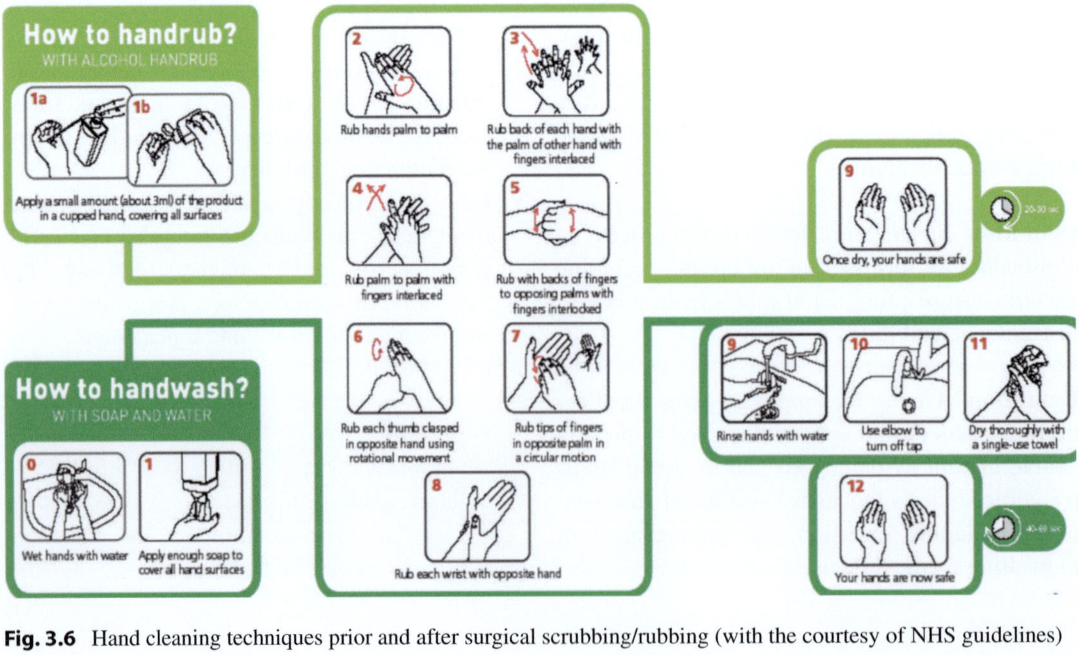

Fig. 3.6 Hand cleaning techniques prior and after surgical scrubbing/rubbing (with the courtesy of NHS guidelines)

Important!
Do not scrub if you have cuts, sores, abrasions, weeping dermatitis, or fresh tattoos on exposed skin as these can harbor microorganisms.

Once all these aspects are encountered, operators should proceed to hand scrub their hands and arms according to the institutional guidelines.

Surgical Hand Antisepsis

As for hand hygiene, two types of procedures are commonly used in healthcare setting prior insertion of a vascular access device (WHO 2009).

Surgical Hand Scrub with Soap and Water

Table 3.1 Hand scrub with medicated soap and water

Steps [3]	Information
Turn on water and start timing	Regulate water temperature ➔ warm water is recommended
Rinse hands and forearms under running water	Clean subungueal areas of both hands under running water using a disposable nail file. Nail brushes are not recommended as they damage the skin
Apply scrub solution to wet hands and forearms	A good amount of soap is required to create lather for a 3–5 min scrub
Rub hands palm to palm, right palm over left dorsum with fingers interlaced, back of fingers to opposing palms, each thumb clasped in the opposite palm with a rotating motion	For each side, consider four surfaces for each finger, thumb, and hand
Scrub the forearms, using up-and-down motion considering four planes. Wash each side from wrist to elbow for 1 min	Always keep hands above elbows ➔ avoids microorganisms to slide off the hands into the sink
Repeat the entire process on the other side	Use an equal amount of time to wash each hand
Rinse hands and arms under running water in one direction only, from fingertips to elbow	Always keep hands raised ➔ this allows all the soap to be rinsed off from cleanest to dirtiest areas
Proceed to the operating theater ensuring hands are kept away from the body and above waist level	This step prevents contamination of the hands and adheres to the principles of sterile technique
Dry hands with a sterile towel following aseptic technique	Start drying at the fingertips and working down toward the forearms using a dabbing motion

Important!
Always keep hands higher than the forearm during hand scrub ➔ avoids recontamination of the hands from water flowing down from the elbows.
Avoid touching the faucet or other contaminated surfaces ➔ if the hand touches anything at any time, the scrub must be lengthened by 1 min for the area that has been contaminated.

Keep the surgical or interventional attire dry since the gown cannot be donned over wet or damp material ➔ risk of contamination of the gown by strike-through moisture.
Dry hands thoroughly using a sterile towel ➔ avoid developing moisture.

Surgical Alcohol-Based Hand Rub (ABHR)
Alcohol-based waterless hand rub (Fig. 3.7) is extremely effective at reducing hand microorganisms and can replace surgical scrub with soap and water unless the hands are visibly soiled [4, 5]. The advantages of ABHRs include the following:

- Less time-consuming
- Remove the majority of germs, including viruses
- Easy to use and access (also before and after patient contact)
- Better skin tolerability

After rubbing forearms (same steps as Table 3.1), make meticulous attention to the following steps to scrub both hands (Fig. 3.7b):

- Apply a palm full of product in cupped hand and cover all surfaces.
- Rub hands palm to palm.
- Rub right palm over left dorsum with fingers interlaced and vice versa.
- Rub hands palm to palm with fingers interlaced.
- Rub backs of fingers to opposing palms with fingers interlocked.
- Perform rotational rubbing of left thumb clasped in right palm and vice versa.
- Perform rotational rubbing, backwards and forwards with clasped fingers of right hand in left palm and vice versa.
- Allow to air-dry. Once dry, your hands are ready for your gloves.

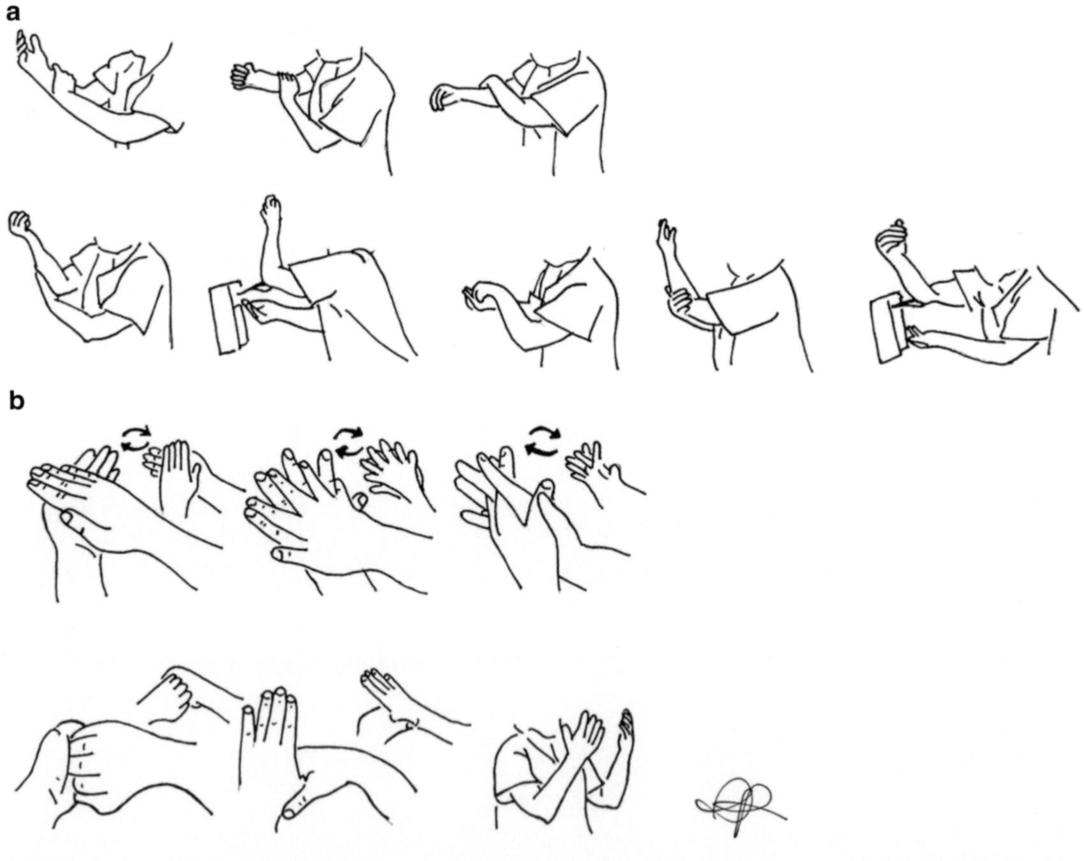

Fig. 3.7 (**a**) Hand rub technique: the steps are depicted from left to right starting from the forearms to conclude with the hand extremities bilaterally. (**b**) Continuation of hand rub technique: the steps for both hands and fingers are depicted from left to right and must be repeated bilaterally for the same amount of time

Both are safe and effective methods to prevent surgical site infections (SSI), although WHO guidelines advocate a slight preference for the use of waterless cleansing alcohol-based formulas, which demonstrate higher antibacterial efficacy. In fact, products containing high concentrations of alcohol (60–90%) provide such a rapid and effective reduction of the resident skin flora, that bacteria regrowth requires up to 6 h to rebuild. These advantages along with rapid action, time savings, less side effects, and low risk of recontamination clearly promote the use of presurgical ABHR in place of soap and water when hands are not visibly soiled [4].

Once surgical hand preparation is done, the next steps include donning sterile gown and gloves.

Gowning

- Always don sterile gown prior to gloves
- Scrubbed personnel gowns are folded on a separate table or surface waist height, away from the main sterile field

Steps:

1. Reach and lift the folded gown directly upward. Do not touch the wrapper and ensure the gown remains folded until after stepping back from the gown table into an unobstructed area.
2. Holding the folded gown like a book by its binding, carefully locate the neckline and armholes.
3. Hold the inside front of the gown just at the armholes with both hands and let the gown unfold, keeping the inside of the gown toward the body and the hands in the armholes. Do not touch the outside of the gown with bare hands. If the top of the gown drops inadvertently, consider it contaminated. Discard and have a new gown pack opened.
4. Slip both arms into the armholes simultaneously moving them in an outward motion as the gown and its sleeves unfold, keeping both hands covered.
5. The circulating personnel stands behind the scrubbed personnel and brings the gown over the shoulders by reaching inside to the shoulder and arm seams. The gown is pulled on, leaving the cuffs of the sleeves extended over the hands. The back of the gown is securely tied at the waist first, followed by the neckline.
6. If the gown is a wrap-around style, the sterile flap to cover the back is not touched until the scrubbed personnel has donned gloves or by use of a sterile item handed to circulating personnel.

Warning!
The neckline, shoulders, under arms, sleeve cuffs, and the back are considered unsterile!

Gloving

- Always examine sterile glove packaging for expiry date, intactness, and tears. The package should be dry (Table 3.2).
- Choose the right size and make sure they are tight enough so that object manipulation and gestures are easy to perform.
- Gather all supplies and prepare your patient for the procedure prior to applying gloves.
- Always don sterile gloves after putting on sterile surgical gown.
- Hands must be washed before and after any procedure.

Important!
Ensure the patient does not have a latex allergy prior to applying sterile gloves, e.g., people who had many surgeries (10+), people often exposed to natural rubber latex, and people with other allergies.

The aforementioned technique is called "closed gloving," in which the hands are not extended from the sleeves and cuffs when the gown is donned and both sterile gown and gloves

Table 3.2 Closed gloving technique

Steps [3, 6]	Information
Inspect packaging for sterility	Removal of the outer packaging (nonsterile) must be done by an assistant prior to starting the procedure. The inner (sterile) package is placed on a sterile surface
Open the two sides like a book by grasping the lower inner corners of the bottom fold. Lift both corners open and fold under at the same time to keep the wrapper open 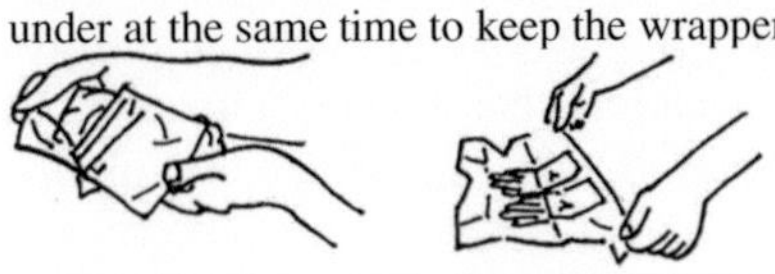	Prevent the package from closing during the gloving process. Right hand glove is on the right, left on the left
Extend the dominant forearm with the palm upward. Grasp the glove cuff with the fingertips of the opposite hand, which is still covered by the sleeve 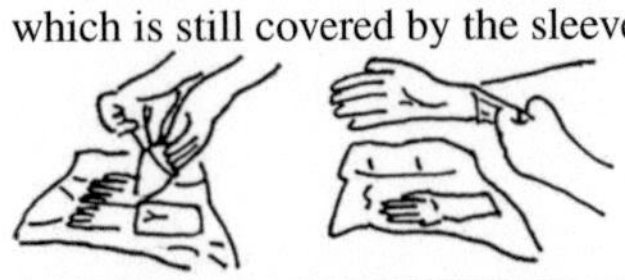	This way only the sterile gown touches the sterile glove. Start with dominant hand with palm facing upward
Slip hand into the glove and pull the cuff over to unroll glove and completely cover the dominant hand and sleeve cuff	Adjust gloves if necessary. Always cover gown cuffs to avoid contamination or skin exposure
Using the gloved hand, open the remaining glove from underneath the cuff and slide hands and fingers of nondominant hand in the glove 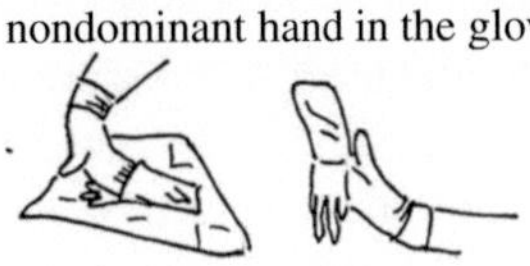	The dominant hand glove should only touch the sterile portion of the remnant glove. Sterile areas can only touch sterile areas 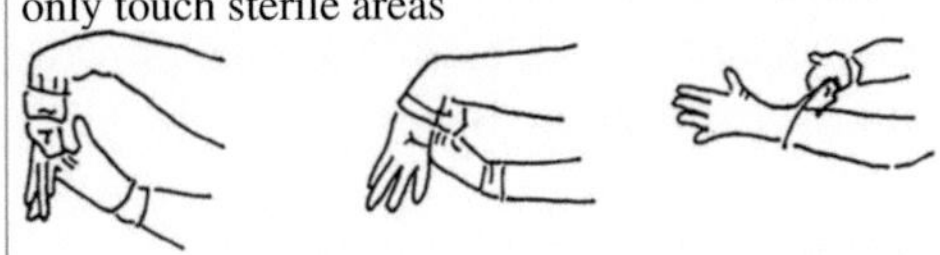
Keep fingers interlocked away from the gown 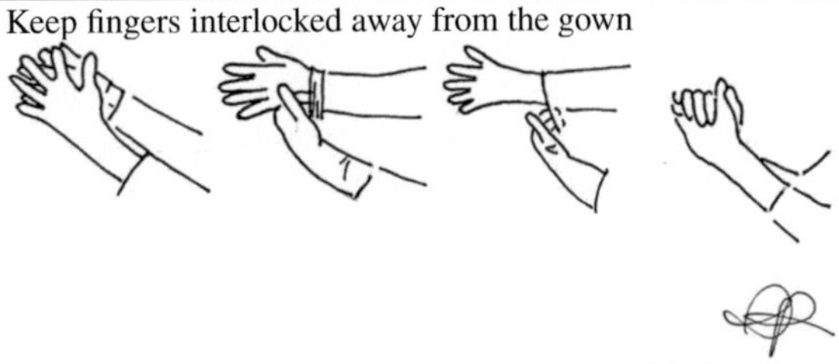	Always keep hands above waist level and below shoulders (see Fig. 3.8) ➔ prevents accidental touching of nonsterile objects

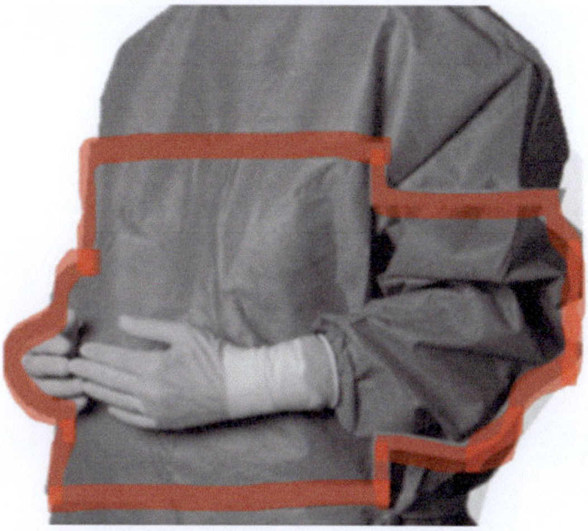

Fig. 3.8 Sterile area and posture after gowning and gloving. Gowns are only considered sterile in the front from the armpit to the level of the sterile field and sleeves from 5 cm above the elbow to cuff (inside the red area)

are handed for each member of the team in a manner to maintain sterility. It differs from the "open gloving" process (Fig. 3.9), meaning the scrubbed person's hands slide all the way through the gown sleeves and cuffs prior to donning gloves.

> **Important!**
> Keep gown cuffs well over hands!
> Gown cuffs are considered unsterile and are to be covered completely by sterile gloves for the following reasons:
>
> - Potential collection of moisture
> - Not effective barrier
> - Contamination while gowning when hands pass through

Glove Removal

To remove sterile gloves, grasp the outside of the cuff at the palm side of the glove with the fingers of the opposite hand and peel it back, rolling it inside out and keeping it in the gloved hand. Remove the other glove by grasping it from the inner cuff palm side with the fingers of the ungloved hand. Remove the glove by turning it inside out entirely and discard them both. To conclude, perform hand hygiene to remove powder and prevent potential contamination from pinholes in the gloves (Fig. 3.10).

> **Overview. Tips for Maintaining Sterility**
> Gloves should always cover wrists and sleeves of sterile gown.
> Avoid contamination by keeping hands and fingers in front of you, interlaced, and above waist level.
> Refrain from touching surfaces, nonsterile items, or adjusting the mask with gloves.
> Any hole or tear in the sterile gloves requires immediate removal and changing.

Preparation for CVC Insertion

The sterile field should be prepared right before the procedure, since the higher time it is exposed to the air, the higher the risk of contamination from airborne microbes. Before opening any furniture, all packages' integrity and expiry date must be checked to ensure that anything contaminated or potentially contaminated gets onto the sterile field. The back table pack is always the first supply to be opened; it allows to cover the back table with a sterile drape where all the other supplies could be opened onto and setup. Opening supplies onto the sterile field also requires appropriate technique: first, unwrap the front flap and then the sides, the inside should not slide near the edges of the package, and items should be flipped onto the table without exposing the arms over the sterile field. Finally, open gowns and gloves for all the operators, preferably on the mayo stand, using the gown wrapper as a sterile field. After surgical scrub, the operator should wear a sterile gown and gloves using the appropriate technique.

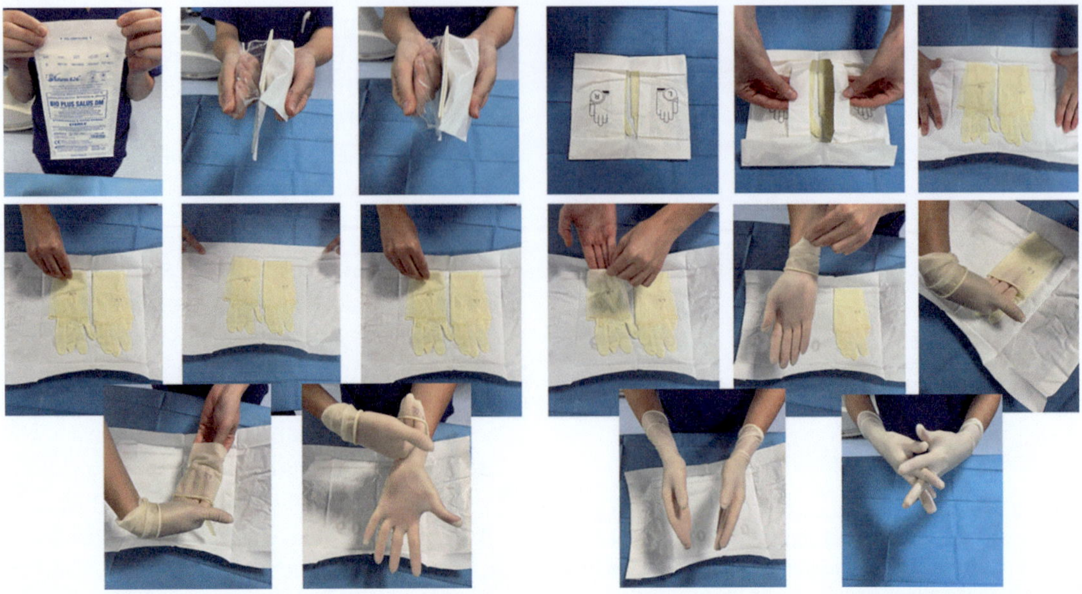

Fig. 3.9 Don sterile gloves: steps from left to right. The skin of the healthcare worker remains exclusively in contact with the inner surface of the glove. Donning surgical sterile gloves at the time of intervention follows these same steps expect that it is performed after wearing sterile gown and prior surgical hand scrubbing/rubbing

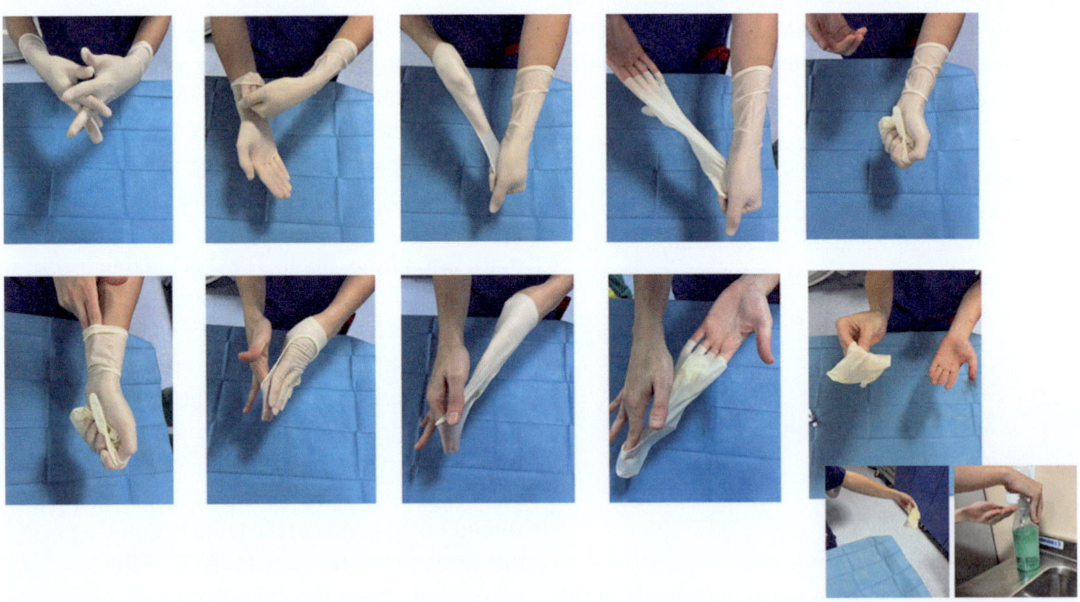

Fig. 3.10 Sterile glove removal: steps to be followed from left to right. Always perform hand hygiene afterwards. If wearing sterile gown, perform the same steps whilst at the end pull off and doff the gown together with the gloves

Key Principles

- Only sterile items are allowed within the sterile field.
- Check each item expiry date.
- Discard any package being wet, dropped, found in unmonitored areas, or showing evidence of crushing, perforations, or holes.

Equipment and Supplies

- Sterile CVC kit (including catheter, guidewire, dilator, introducer needle, scalpel, forceps, and sutures)
- Sterile gloves and gown
- Nonsterile mask and cap
- Antiseptic solution (e.g., chlorhexidine or povidone-iodine)
- Sterile drapes and dressings
- Sterile ultrasound probe cover (if using ultrasound guidance)
- Sterile saline solution, needles, and syringes

Preparing the Insertion Site

When the back table and operators are prepped in sterile gown and gloves, it is time to prepare the surgical field. Percutaneous procedures carry an intrinsic risk of contamination from pathogenic microorganisms and infection. For this reason, maximal barrier precautions during insertion are mandatory. An antimicrobial agent is used to reduce the microbial count with the broader range of germicidal action, according to eventual patient allergies or sensitivities. Hair removal should accurately be performed before disinfection.

Skin Antisepsis

- Antiseptic agents: use an antiseptic solution such as chlorhexidine gluconate, povidone-iodine, or alcohol-based preparations to the skin at the insertion site ➔ *2% chlorhexidine in 70% isopropyl alcohol* is often preferred due to its superior and prolonged antimicrobial activity [7].
- Application technique: apply the solution using a back-and-forth friction motion for at least 30 s, allowing the antiseptic to air-dry completely before proceeding with catheter insertion (do not blow or blot dry!).

Summary

Use a chlorhexidine-containing solution for skin preparation in adults, infants, and children (lower infection rate and only 30 s to be effective vs. 90 s with povidone-iodine).

For neonates, determine the use of chlorhexidine-containing solutions for skin preparation based on clinical judgment and institutional protocol.

If there is a contraindication to chlorhexidine, povidone-iodine or alcohol may be used.

Unless contraindicated, use skin preparation solutions containing alcohol.

Draping

Cover the area with sterile small and full-body drapes to create a large sterile field around the insertion site ➔ once the sterile drape is placed, it must not be moved or rearranged.

Warning!

Do not touch skin with gloved hands or with the catheter!

Establishing a Sterile Field

- Use sterile drapes to cover surfaces or operative fields.
- Surgical drapes are considered sterile only at table level; the edges of the drape below the working surface are not.

- Any item that is handed off the table is considered unsterile (e.g., tubing).
- Ensure all items that will contact the catheter insertion site or catheter pathway remain within the sterile field.
- The edges of packages are considered unsterile; prevent wrapper from touching the sterile field or package contents.
- Keep sterile surfaces clean and dry ➔ moisture can cause strike-through and contaminate the sterile field [3].

Dispensing Sterile Items

- Open supplies as close to possible to the surgical starting time.
- Minimize handling sterile equipment to reduce contamination.
- Check packages' integrity, chemical indicators, and expiry dates.
- The sterile boundary of a peel-open package is the inner edge.
- Do not rip or torn peel pouches which must be gently peeled backwards.
- Expose the contents so the scrubbed personnel can remove the item from the wrapper by grasping it with hands or forceps.
- Do not flip, shake, or drop items onto the sterile field.

> **Warning!**
> These motions create air turbulence, contamination, and potential damage!

Pour sterile solutions into a sterile receptacle; this must be placed away from the table avoiding the need for the assistant to reach across the sterile field.

Maintaining a Sterile Field

- Circulating personnel must not touch or reach over sterile items or areas.
- Scrubbed personnel should avoid touching nonsterile surfaces or objects during the procedure.
- If the circulating personnel opens a sterile pack, the wrap is opened first away from the circulating personnel to prevent contamination.
- Sterile personnel must stay close to the sterile field and never turn their back on the sterile field.
- If sterile personnel change position, they can move face to face or back to back.

> **Warning!**
> Do not leave open sterile supplies unattended and monitor them continuously.

Insertion Process

- Ultrasound guidance: use of sterile gel and sterile probe cover during insertion to visualize the target vein and surrounding structures, which enhances the accuracy of catheter placement and reduces the risk of complications
- Sterile technique during insertion: maintaining sterility throughout the insertion process by avoiding contact with nonsterile surfaces and ensuring that all movements and adjustments are performed within the sterile field
  - Anesthetize the insertion site with sterile technique
  - Insert the introducer needle and guidewire, followed by the dilator, maintaining sterility throughout

- Insert the catheter over the guidewire into the central vein
- Secure the catheter with sutures and apply a sterile dressing

Catheter Care and Maintenance

Postinsertion Catheter Site Care

- Dressing: cover the insertion site with a sterile, transparent, semipermeable dressing
- Dressing changes: perform routine dressing changes or immediately replace the dressings when they become wet, visibly soiled, or loose

> **Important!**
> Every 7 days for transparent dressings, every 48 h for gauze dressings, and on a daily basis for ICU patients.

Catheter Maintenance

- Hand hygiene: always comply to hand hygiene requirements before handling the catheter or accessing the line
- Aseptic access: use sterile technique when accessing the catheter for blood draws, medication administration, or flushing
  - Scrub the access port or hub with friction immediately prior to each use with an appropriate antiseptic (chlorhexidine, povidone-iodine, an iodophor, or 70% alcohol)
  - Use only sterile devices to access catheters

> **Important!**
> Immediately replace dressings that are wet, soiled, or dislodged!

- Antiseptic cap: use antiseptic caps or devices on catheter hubs when not in use to prevent contamination
- Flushing protocols: regularly flush the catheter with saline or heparinized saline to maintain patency and prevent clot formation, following institution-specific protocols for flushing frequency and technique

Monitoring for Infection

- Regularly inspect the insertion site for signs of infection, such as redness, swelling, or discharge
- Monitor the patient for systemic signs of infection, such as fever or chills
- Ensure that the dressing remains intact and secured
- Replace the catheter if infection is suspected or confirmed
- Promptly remove central lines when no longer deemed clinically necessary

Education and Training

Ensuring that healthcare providers are adequately trained in sterilization and aseptic techniques is essential for preventing infections during CVC.

- Competency training: regular training sessions and competency assessments for healthcare professionals involved in CVC placement and maintenance
- Continuous education: keeping staff updated on the latest guidelines and best practices for aseptic technique and infection prevention

Summary of the Five Key Points of CVC Bundle [6]

Hand hygiene
Maximal barrier precautions before and during insertion (mask, cap, gown, sterile gloves, and drapes)
Aseptic technique
Site selection considering individual patient characteristics
Regular maintenance of catheter

Conclusions

Adhering to stringent sterilization and aseptic techniques is essential to prevent infections related to central venous catheterization. By following the outlined protocols for preparation, insertion, and maintenance, healthcare providers can significantly reduce the risk of catheter-related bloodstream infections, thereby ensuring safer patient outcomes. Ensuring proper training and ongoing education for all healthcare personnel involved in CVC procedures is essential for sustaining high standards of patient care and safety.

References

1. Tennant KRCL. Sterile technique. StatPearls; 2024.
2. World Health Organization. Patient Safety. WHO guidelines on hand hygiene in health care: first global patient safety challenge clean care is safer care. WHO; 2009. 262 p.
3. Doyle G, McCutcheon J. Clinical procedures for safer patient care. BCcampus; 2015.
4. O'Grady NP, Alexander M, Burns LA, Dellinger EP, Garland J, Heard SO, et al. Guidelines for the prevention of intravascular catheter-related infections. Clin Infect Dis. 2011;52(9):e162.
5. The 2016 Infusion Therapy Standards [Internet]. 2017. Available from: www.homehealthcarenow.org.
6. Moureau NL. Vessel health and preservation: the right approach for vascular access. Springer International Publishing; 2019. p. 1–303.
7. Practice guidelines for Central Venous Access 2020: an updated report by the American Society of Anesthesiologists Task Force on Central Venous Access. Anesthesiology. 2020;132(1):8–43.

4 Access Techniques

Boris Tufegdzic and Massimo Lamperti

Introduction

Central venous cannulation (CVC) is a commonly performed procedure that involves percutaneously placing a vascular catheter within the lumen of a major, high-flowing vein of the abdomen or thorax. This catheter can facilitate the administration of fluids, blood products, medications, nutritional support, and long-term vascular access. It is a relatively standard procedure in many branches of medicine, particularly in anaesthesia and intensive care units.

Central venous cannulation is indicated when peripheral venous access is unavailable or not recommended. Where to place a central line is typically based on clinical indicators or individual clinician experience and preference. Knowledge of the vascular system is essential for providing care to the patient for CVC. While the evidence does not suggest only one area for placement, each location has known risks and benefits.

The placement of a central venous catheter was first described in 1929 [1] by 25-year-old Werner Forssmann, a German surgical resident, who punctured his left antecubital vein and passed a 4-Fr ureteric catheter 35 cm centrally. From its modest beginning in 1929 to today, central venous access has matured to become an essential component of modern medical care. Improvements in catheter materials and properties, safety features, and device options have made this an ever-evolving technology field.

A site for central venous cannulation and catheter/device selection requires a collaborative approach between healthcare team members and the patient. Considerations include patient assessment, treatment type, treatment duration, type of access device, and patient's values and preferences. Device selection is guided by the principles of the least invasive, fewest lumens, and smallest gauge catheter appropriate for the treatment. The device should last for the duration of the patient's required treatment.

Preparation for Central Venous Cannulation

Patient Assessment, Education, and Informed Consent

Patient assessment includes both health history and physical assessment. Medical conditions of concern, besides allergy status, include coagulation status, diabetes, renal disease, trauma, and previous central venous cannulation. Other conditions to note are previous arm, neck, or chest trauma; surgery; or radiation. Physical assessment is needed for circulatory status, lymphedema, and skin integrity.

B. Tufegdzic · M. Lamperti (✉)
Anesthesiology Division, Cleveland Clinic Abu Dhabi, Abu Dhabi, UAE

R. Lanocita, M. Lamperti (eds.), *Practical Guide to Central Venous Cannulation*,
https://doi.org/10.1007/978-3-031-90326-7_4

Before venous cannulation, the risks and benefits of the procedure should be reviewed. Written consent should be obtained from the patient, patient family, or legal representative.

Explaining the reasons for the CVC and the procedure will allay fears and help the patient participate as much as possible. Engaging the patient and the family in all aspects of care, particularly infection prevention and maintenance of the central venous catheter, will help improve patient outcomes.

Ultrasound Pre-procedural Assessment

The ultrasound (US) pre-procedural assessment of all peripheral and central veins is highly recommended. This allows for the identification of vessels which may be challenging to puncture because they are either small, collapsed during breathing, or altered by anatomical and pathological variations. Pre-procedural ultrasound evaluation is important for defining the preferable access site, minimising insertion-related risks, and preventing post-insertion-related complications. It is important to try to predict future needs for vascular access as poor prospective management can lead to interruptions in therapy, exhaustion of the peripheral vasculature, and the psychological trauma of repeated procedures.

Different protocols are used in daily clinical practice. Depending on the planned approach for central venous cannulation, we can use the rapid central vein assessment protocol (RaCeVA), rapid femoral vein assessment protocol (RaFeVA), or rapid peripheral vein assessment protocol (RaPeVA). The ultrasound-based evaluation of all peripheral and central veins should always be performed bilaterally using the RaPeVA, RaCeVA, and RaFeVA.

Rapid Central Vein Assessment (RaCeVA) Protocol

Pre-procedural supra/infra-clavicular area scanning is performed according to the rapid central vein assessment (RaCeVA) protocol [2]. RaCeVA should be performed before a centrally inserted central catheter, helping the operator to consider systematically all possible venous options and to rule out potential anatomic or pathological alterations of the vein that the catheter will occupy.

RaCeVA protocol is consistent with seven steps starting at the mid-neck region, with the transducer in a transverse position over the anterior neck, perpendicular to the skin. In step 2, the transducer will slide caudally still in a transverse position, but it is located in the lower neck, in the suprasternal area. The next step will include tilting the transducer from a perpendicular to a frontal plane, parallel to the clavicle, close (and lateral) to the sternal notch. The probe further slides laterally in the supraclavicular area while still in a frontal plane, allowing the visualisation of the subclavian vein on the long axis, just behind the clavicle. Step 5 moves the probe to the infraclavicular area, parallel to the clavicle (perpendicular to the deltopectoral groove), and transverse to the thoracic wall. Kept in the same place, the probe will be gently rotated on its axis. It is now longitudinal and perpendicular to the thoracic wall, parallel to the deltopectoral groove. In the last step, pleural function assessment should be done in the pre-insertion phase (Table 4.1).

Table 4.1 The seven steps of the rapid central vein assessment (RaCeVA)

	Transducer position	Structures to be assessed
Step 1	Mid-neck (transverse)	Internal jugular vein Carotid artery
Step 2	Base of neck (transverse)	Internal jugular vein Carotid artery Subclavian artery
Step 3	Sternoclavicular (transverse)	Internal jugular vein Brachiocephalic vein
Step 4	Supraclavicular (longitudinal)	Subclavian vein Subclavian artery External jugular vein
Step 5	Infraclavicular (transverse)	Axillary vein Axillary artery Cephalic vein
Step 6	Infraclavicular (longitudinal)	Axillary vein Axillary artery
Step 7	Sliding lung (longitudinal)	Pleura (anterior chest wall)

Rapid Femoral Vein Assessment (RaFeVA) Protocol

Before a femorally inserted central catheter, the veins of the lower extremities are scanned according to the RaFeVA protocol [3]. The protocol consists of seven steps, considering the different possible visualisations of the vessels (along the short, long, or oblique axes) and proposing different venipuncture techniques (out-of-plane and in-plane).

For method, the user should start with the RaFeVA protocol at the inguinal groove with the probe in a transverse position, perpendicular to the skin. Identify the common femoral artery (CFA) and the common femoral vein (CFV), both on the short axis. Switch to visualise the transition between the CFV and the external iliac vein in the long axis. After returning to a short-axis view, move the probe caudally, to visualise the CFA, CFV, and saphenous vein (SV), in the short-axis view. In the next step, slide the probe downward, far from the groin, still in a transverse view, to visualise the superficial femoral artery (SFA), the deep femoral artery (DFA), and the CFV, all in the short axis. At the end, slide the probe caudally, towards mid-thigh, to visualise the SFA and the SFV in the short- and oblique-axis view (Table 4.2).

Table 4.2 The seven steps of the rapid femoral vein assessment (RaFeVA) protocol

	Transducer position	Structures to be assessed
Step 1	Short axis	Common femoral artery Common femoral vein
Step 2	Long axis	Common femoral vein External iliac vein
Step 3	Short axis	Common femoral artery Common femoral vein Saphenous vein
Step 4	Short axis	Superficial femoral artery Deep femoral artery Common femoral vein
Step 5	Short axis	Superficial femoral artery Deep femoral artery Superficial femoral vein Deep femoral vein
Step 6	Short axis	Superficial femoral artery Superficial femoral vein
Step 7	Oblique axis	Superficial femoral artery Superficial femoral vein

Rapid Peripheral Vein Assessment (RaPeVA) Protocol

The rapid peripheral vein assessment (RaPeVA) [4] is the protocol developed to collect relevant anatomical information before positioning a peripherally inserted central catheter (PICC). It guides the operator in selecting the most appropriate vein to be accessed, on a rational and well-informed, by assessing calibre and collapsibility, depth, patency, and anatomic relationships with sensitive structures. The transducer is placed transverse to the axis of the limb and perpendicular to the skin to obtain an optimal panoramic view of the veins in their relationship to other structures, importantly arteries and nerves.

The seven steps of RaPeVA are performed in the following systematic approach; after visualisation of the cephalic vein at the antecubital fossa, the probe is moved from the radial side to the ulnar side, until the artery and brachial veins are identified and the confluence between the antecubital vein and basilic vein is seen. In the next step, sliding the probe upwards, identification of the basilic vein along the bicipital-humeral groove will be done together with an examination of the nerve-vascular bundle of the arm. Then, we will visualise the cephalic vein, moving the transducer laterally over the biceps muscle, and examine the axillary vein in the infraclavicular area and the internal jugular, subclavian, and brachiocephalic vein in the supraclavicular region (Table 4.3).

Table 4.3 The seven steps of the rapid peripheral vein assessment (RaPeVA) protocol

	Structures to be assessed
Step 1	Cephalic vein at the antecubital fossa
Step 2	Artery and brachial veins and of the confluence between the antecubital vein and the basilic vein
Step 3	Basilic vein in the bicipital-humeral groove
Step 4	Nerve-vascular bundle of the arm
Step 5	Cephalic vein over the biceps muscle
Step 6	Axillary vein in the infraclavicular area
Step 7	Internal jugular, the subclavian, and the brachiocephalic vein in the supraclavicular area

Laboratory Tests

In less urgent situations, it is a common practice to evaluate coagulation parameters (platelet count and international normalised ratio/prothrombin time) and correct abnormalities (target INR <1.5, PTT <40, platelets >50,000) before line insertion. However, no randomised studies exist to support this approach. A systematic review, studying the risk of complications following central venous line placement in patients with moderate-to-severe coagulopathy and thrombocytopenia, revealed that the incidence of major bleeding complications is low, and evidence supporting the correction of coagulopathy before central venous line placement is lacking [5]. In reality, many CVCs can be safely placed in coagulopathic patients, and the likelihood of mechanical complications depends more on the skill and experience of the operator in using ultrasound for guidance than on any single laboratory value [6].

Patient Positioning

The patient should be in an anatomically advantageous position for the procedure. The patient should be placed in the Trendelenburg position for the internal jugular and subclavian veins to increase the vessel's size and improve the chance of first-pass success. For a subclavian approach, the patient's arm should be adducted and the head neutral, or only slightly to the contralateral side to expose the internal jugular vein but not to cause overlap with the carotid artery.

For femoral vein access, the patient should be in a supine position. The target leg is abducted and externally rotated 15° to open the femoral triangle. Elevation of the buttock with rolled sheets or a firm pillow facilitates exposure in some patients. Head-up positioning, reverse Trendelenburg, may augment the cross-sectional area of the femoral vein, but the effect is not universal.

Adjust the bed height and remove clothing, jewellery, and any non-essential equipment that may impede the preparation of a clear sterile field.

Preparation for the Procedure

When the assistant is present and the patient is ready, perform hand hygiene and don the sterile personal protective equipment. Open the sterile equipment, creating a "sterile field". Prepare the central venous catheter by attaching saline locks with saline flushes and flushing all ports to ensure no equipment issues. Remove the saline lock from the most distal port (Fig. 4.1). Place the sterile drape over the patient, with the access point over the procedure site.

To prepare the ultrasound probe, have an assistant dispense enough acoustic gel to cover the transducer surface. Then, have the assistant carefully feed the probe into a sterile transducer sheath while extending the sheath away from you over the length of the probe cable. Eliminate any wrinkles or air bubbles that appear between the transducer and the sheath to ensure secure acoustic coupling. Secure the sheath around the transducer using sterile rubber bands or plastic clips. Apply a small amount of sterile ultrasound gel to the covered ultrasound probe or the patient's skin. Because the sterile ultrasound probe is used intermittently throughout the procedure, you should identify a convenient sterile area where the probe can be placed when not in use (Fig. 4.2) [7].

Ensure that all equipment is within reach before initiating the procedure (Fig. 4.3).

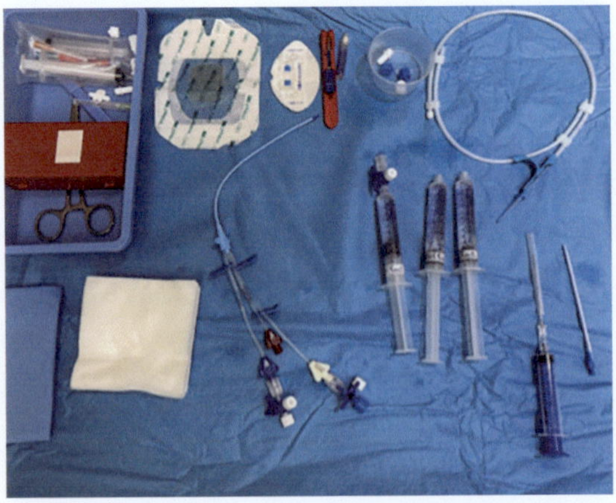

Fig. 4.1 Preparation for the procedure—sterile field

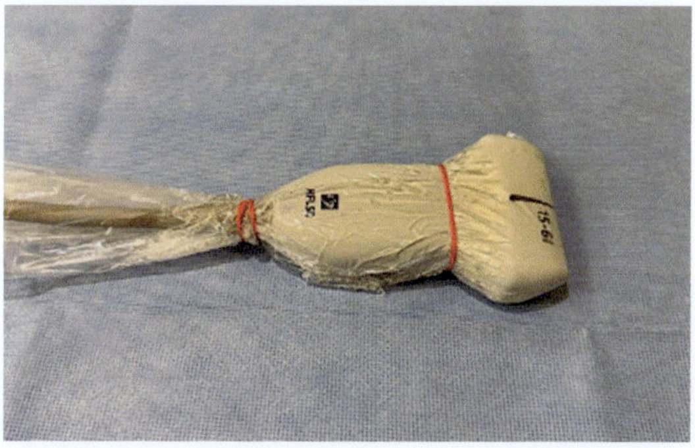

Fig. 4.2 Preparation for the procedure—ultrasound probe

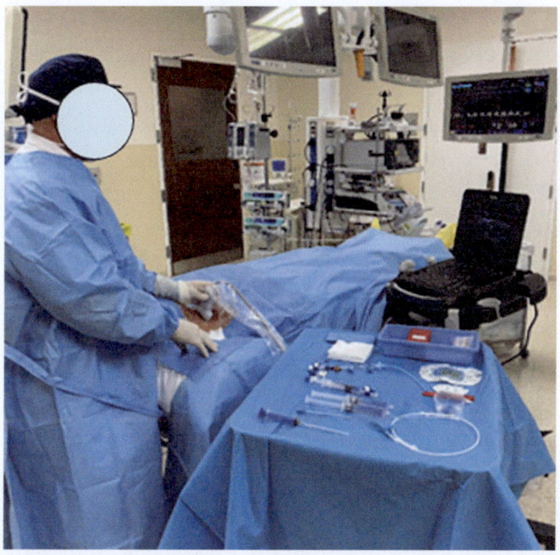

Fig. 4.3 Proceduralist orientation during CVC

Before any medical procedure, the proceduralist should perform a "time out" with theatre staff to confirm that the team is with the right patient and performing the correct procedure at the right site.

Unless the patient is under general anaesthesia or deeply sedated, use a 25-gauge needle to infiltrate the skin with a local anaesthetic, such as 1% or 2% lidocaine.

Insertion of a Central Venous Catheter

Where to place a central line is typically based on clinical parameters and individual clinician experience and preference. Traditionally, CVC placement was performed using landmark techniques based on the knowledge of anatomic structures and palpation of arteries next to the veins. These landmark techniques cannot account for anatomic variations or venous thromboses, especially in oncologic and critically ill patients. This could make central venous catheter placement impossible or dangerous. In contrast, ultrasound can be used to easily visualise anatomic structures and confirm patency of the vein, thus helping to avoid unintended arterial puncture or unsuccessful cannulation. Modern medicine has been remarkably improved using ultrasound for vascular access, significantly improving patient safety, effectiveness, and efficiency.

Landmark Versus Ultrasound

Cochrane systematic reviews and meta-analyses, published in 2015, summarise the current evidence for ultrasound guidance versus anatomic landmark techniques for CVC placement in the internal jugular vein [8], subclavian vein [9], and femoral vein [9] about complications of CVC placement. These Cochrane reviews suggest that there is evidence that ultrasound offers gains in safety and quality during CVC placement in the internal jugular vein. These reviews indicate that ultrasound offers small gains in safety and quality for the subclavian and femoral veins.

Based on the available evidence from clinical studies, several medical society guidelines strongly recommend using ultrasound for CVC placement in the internal jugular vein.

In 2012, a joint guideline from the American Society of Echocardiography and the Society of Cardiovascular Anesthesiologists [10] strongly recommended the use of real-time ultrasound for CVC placement in the internal jugular vein. It was not recommended for the subclavian vein. No recommendation for routine use of US was made for the femoral vein because of insufficient scientific evidence.

In 2016, the Association of Anaesthetists of Great Britain and Ireland [11] also recommended the routine use of ultrasound for CVC placement in the internal jugular vein. The expert group recommends ultrasound use "for all other central venous access sites, but recognises evidence is, at present, limited".

Recent guidelines published in 2020 by the European Society of Anaesthesiology recommend using ultrasound guidance for internal jugular vein cannulation in adults, as it is safer to reduce overall complications. It improves overall and first-time success, reducing the time to puncture and cannulate the vein successfully. The level of evidence was classified as 1B [12].

Ultrasound for CVC Placement

The first reported use of ultrasound to guide central venous access was by Peters in 1982 [13]. Ultrasound probes most applicable for CVC placement are linear array probes with high-frequency transducers (5–15 MHz). These probes usually have a 20–50 mm scanning surface, allowing high-resolution imaging of superficial anatomic structures. 2D imaging is currently the standard technique used for ultrasound-guided central venous access. All ultrasound probes have an index mark (a small physical notch on one side of the probe) that corresponds with an orientation marker on one side of the ultrasound scan sector shown on the screen and thus helps to obtain the correct probe orientation during examination [14].

Ultrasound can be used in different ways to facilitate CVC placement. "Static" ultrasound or "ultrasound-assisted" CVC placement (also called indirect ultrasound) describes a technique using ultrasound before CVC placement to identify the anatomy of the target vein and adjacent anatomic structures (including the patency of the vein and its dimensions and depth from the skin). In contrast, "real-time" ultrasound or ultrasound-guided CVC placement (direct ultrasound) describes a technique of needle advancement and vessel puncture under permanent ultrasound control.

The ultrasound probe can be placed in a transverse position relative to the vessel, resulting in a "short-axis" view on the ultrasound screen, a cross-sectional image of the vessel. A "long-axis" view, or a longitudinal image of the vessel, is obtained by placing the ultrasound probe in a parallel position relative to the vessel's course. Short-axis and long-axis views can be used for US assistance and CVC placement guidance. Additionally, the terms "out-of-plane" and "in-plane" describe the direction of the needle relative to the ultrasound probe.

The short-axis (cross-sectional, transverse) ultrasound view is easy to obtain and better for identifying veins, arteries, and their orientation to each other. Identifying a needle tip in cross-section requires some skill because the needle appears as an echogenic, white dot, and the tip can be distinguished only by the dot's disappearance and reappearance as the needle tip traverses back and forth across the imaging plane. The short-axis view is typically used to determine a suitable venous impalement site and to guide steeply angled (e.g. ≥5°) needle insertions (Fig. 4.4).

The long-axis (longitudinal, in-plane) ultrasound view is technically more challenging to obtain (must keep probe, vein, and needle in one plane), but it shows the needle longitudinally, so the entire needle (including the tip) can be imaged continuously as it approaches and enters the vein; this helps avoid aberrant placement. The long-axis view is helpful when the needle insertion angle is shallow (e.g. in axillary/subclavian cannulations) and to affirm proper longitudinal needle alignment during short-axis insertions (Fig. 4.5).

The oblique orientation of the ultrasound probe may offer improved needle visibility during ultrasound-guided vascular access. The oblique view capitalises on the strengths and minimises

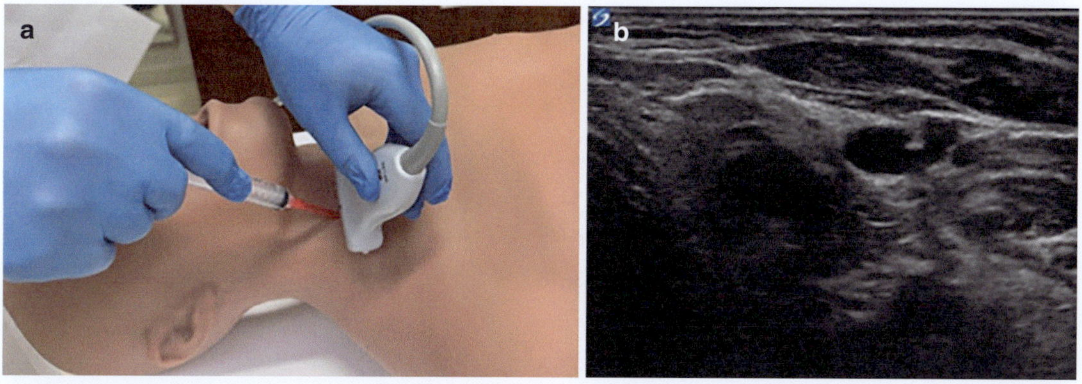

Fig. 4.4 A two-panel image showing a medical procedure. Panel (**a**) depicts a person wearing blue gloves using an ultrasound probe on a mannequin's neck while inserting a needle. Panel (**b**) displays an ultrasound image of the neck area, showing various tissue layers and structures

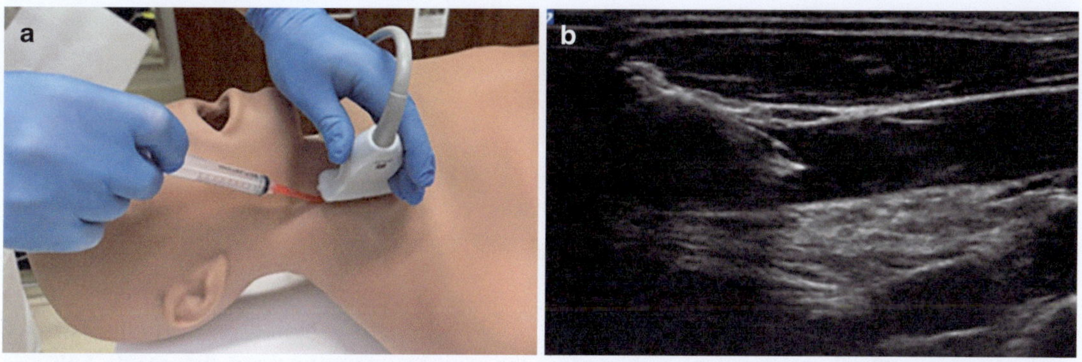

Fig. 4.5 A two-panel image showing a medical procedure. Panel (**a**) depicts a person wearing blue gloves performing an ultrasoundguided procedure on a medical mannequin's neck using a syringe and an ultrasound probe. Panel (**b**) displays an ultrasound image of the neck area, showing tissue layers and structures. The image illustrates the use of ultrasound in medical training and procedures

the weaknesses of the short- and long-axis approaches to yield an optimised venous cannulation approach (Fig. 4.6).

It is essential to understand that the user needs to align the ultrasound and needle plane, containing the needle that appears on the screen as a point (short-axis/out-of-plane) or an echogenic line (long-axis/in-plane) with ring-down artefacts [15].

Seldinger Technique

Various techniques to safely gain access were proposed with the growth in indications for central venous access. Despite these advancements, the procedure has remained relatively unchanged since the advent of the Seldinger technique. It is named after Sven Ivar Seldinger, a Swedish radiologist who introduced the procedure in 1953 [16]. His groundbreaking technique, introduced at the Karolinska Hospital, marked a pivotal moment in medical history.

The Seldinger technique utilises a steel needle to introduce a guidewire into a vessel. The versatility of the Seldinger technique is evident in its wide range of applications across various medical disciplines (but not limited to):

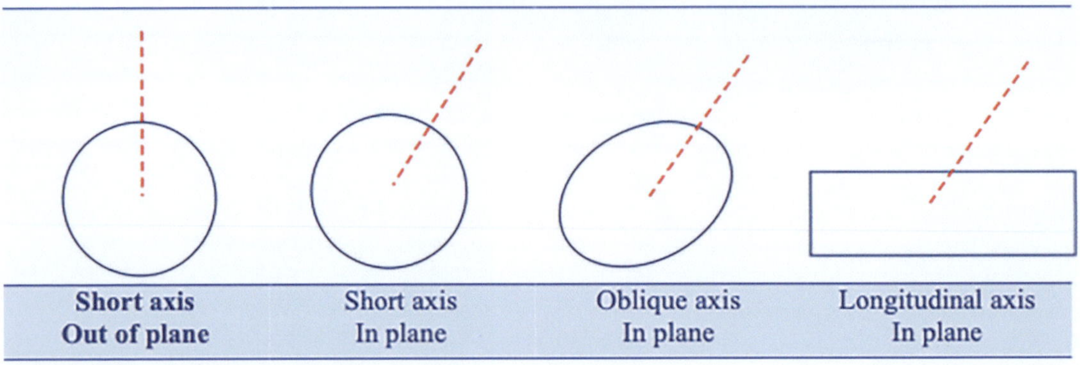

Fig. 4.6 Vessel visualisation and needle-to-ultrasound beam orientation

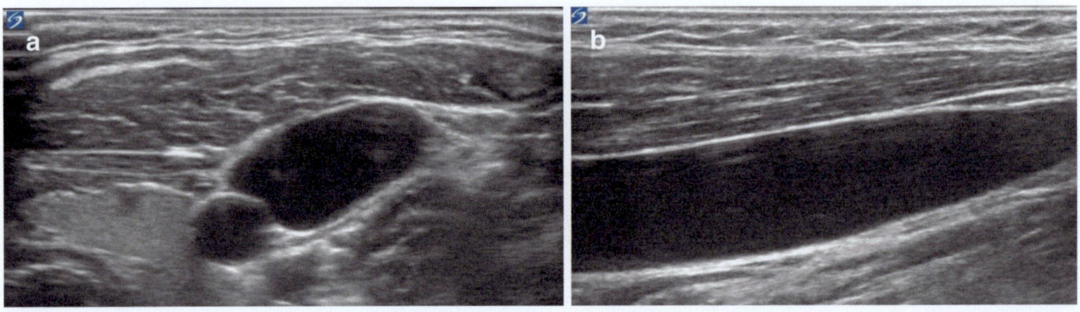

Fig. 4.7 Identify the anatomy of the insertion site and localisation of the vein: (**a**) short-axis view; (**b**) long-axis view

- Venous access for central venous catheters
- Venous or arterial access for cardiology procedures
- Venous or arterial access for interventional radiology procedures
- Insertion of chest tubes and drains
- Insertion of PEG tubes

The following steps will present using the Seldinger technique for central venous cannulation using an ultrasound-guided approach.

After confirming the patency and after the selected vein is prepped and draped, the insertion site should be anaesthetised by injecting local anaesthetic into the subcutaneous tissue sufficient to create a wheel under the skin (Figs. 4.7 and 4.8).

Position the needle bevel facing up on your syringe. Place the introducer needle into the skin at a 45° angle, although this may vary based on the patient's anatomy, and advance towards the selected vein while aspirating with steady pressure (Fig. 4.9).

When a flash of blood appears in the barrel of the syringe, securely grasp the needle hub and hold it motionless. Remove the syringe from the needle hub and briefly let blood flow out to confirm that the blood is venous, dark red, and flowing but not pulsatile. Immediately after, cover the hub with your thumb to stop the blood flow and prevent air embolism.

However, if the blood is bright red and pulsatile (arterial), terminate the procedure. Remove the needle and use 4 × 4 gauze squares for 10 minutes to hold external pressure on the area to decrease bleeding from the puncture site.

Some commercial kits include a syringe with a wire port located on the base of the plunger, allowing the wire to be inserted into the vein (Fig. 4.10).

If the blood is venous, carefully insert the J-curved end of the guidewire into the introducer needle, with the J-curve facing inferiorly in the same direction as the needle bevel. Advance the guidewire through the needle and into the vein. Do not force the wire; it should slide smoothly.

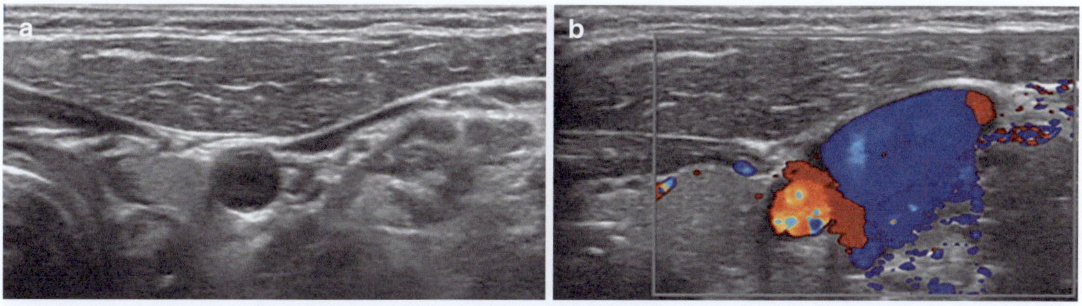

Fig. 4.8 Confirm patency of the vein: (**a**) compression; (**b**) colour Doppler

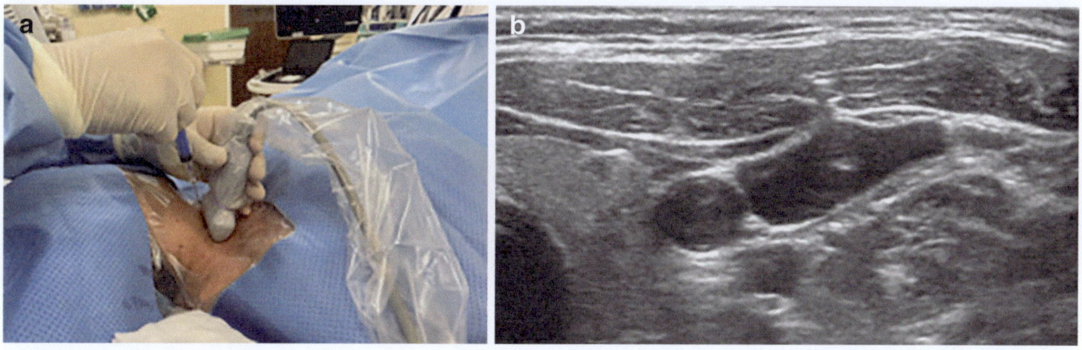

Fig. 4.9 A two-panel image labeled "**a**" and "**b**." Panel "**a**" shows a medical procedure where a healthcare professional, wearing gloves, is using an ultrasound probe on a patient's abdomen, covered with a sterile drape. Panel "**b**" displays an ultrasound image of internal body structures, showing various tissue layers and textures

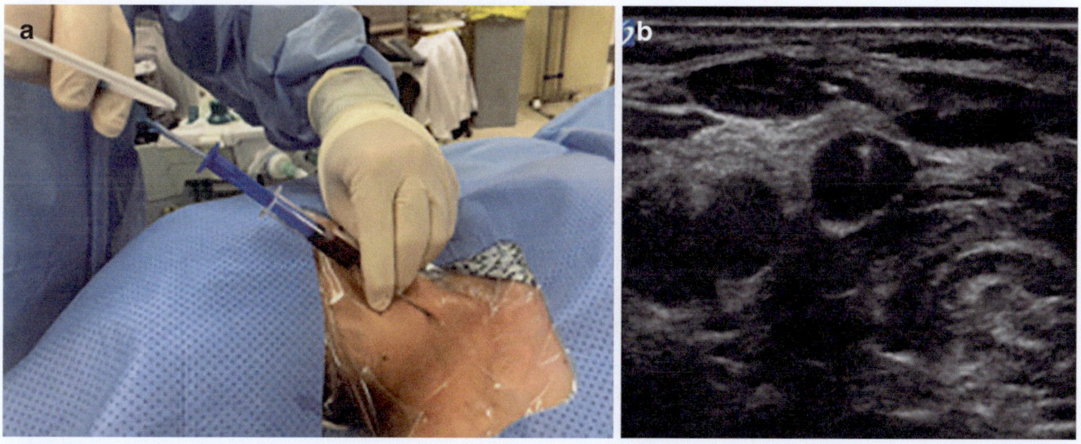

Fig. 4.10 A two-panel image. Panel (**a**) shows a medical procedure where a healthcare professional, wearing gloves and a blue gown, is using a syringe to extract fluid from a patient's abdomen, covered with a sterile drape. Panel (**b**) displays an ultrasound image showing internal structures, likely related to the procedure in panel (**a**). The ultrasound image includes various shades of gray indicating different tissue densities

Advance the wire 15–20 cm or until ectopic heartbeats occur. In case ectopic heartbeats occur, withdraw from this point until ectopy stops.

Stop advancing the guidewire if you feel any resistance as you advance. Try to gently withdraw the wire slightly, rotate it slightly, and then

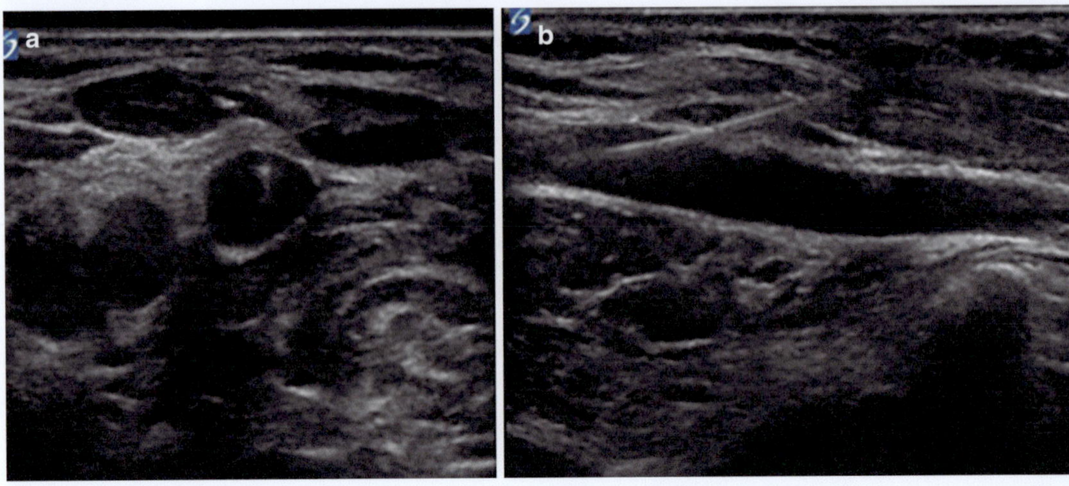

Fig. 4.11 Confirm wire position in the vein: (**a**) short-axis view; (**b**) long-axis view

readvance it, or gently withdraw the wire entirely, re-establish the needle tip within the vein (confirmed by venous blood return), and reinsert the wire.

However, if you feel any resistance as you withdraw the wire, terminate the procedure and withdraw the needle and guidewire together to prevent the needle tip from shearing through the guidewire.

After the guidewire is successfully inserted, the needle is removed (and the syringe is still attached). It is always important to keep control of the guidewire so that it does not completely (Figs. 4.10 and 4.11).

Using the scalpel, make a small stab incision into the skin insertion site, avoiding contact with the guidewire, to enlarge the site and allow it to accommodate the larger diameters of the tissue dilator and the catheter. Maintain your grasp on the wire at all times during the insertion. Although it was previously recommended to use the scalpel to make a small stab incision into the path of the guidewire, using only the skin dilator over the wire will help dilate the soft tissue to the vein, reducing the risk of bleeding and a possible post incisional scar. After removing the dilator, we will likely have increased bleeding from the site due to the dilation. Using gauze and direct, moderate pressure over the cannulation site will decrease bleeding and allow the wire's continued security (Fig. 4.12).

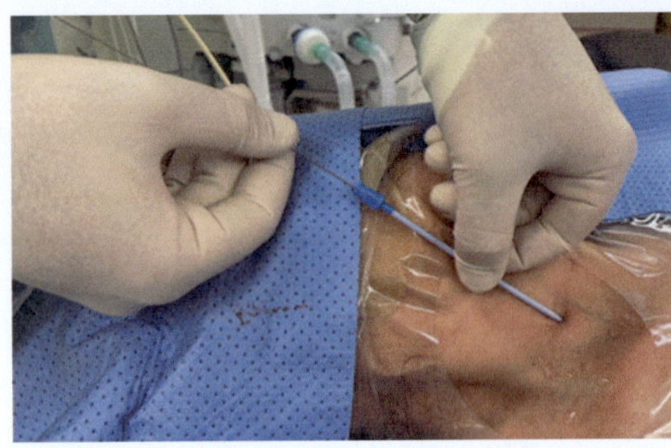

Fig. 4.12 Use the skin dilator over the wire to dilate the soft tissue

After removing the dilator, hold the guidewire fixed at the skin surface, thread the catheter tip over the distal end, and slide the catheter down to the skin surface. The distal end of the guidewire should now be protruding from the port hub. If the distal end of the guidewire is not protruding from the port hub, inch the guidewire outward from the skin surface while holding the catheter tip close to the surface until the guidewire protrudes. In triple-lumen catheters, the wire will emerge from the brown port.

Continue to advance the catheter into the vein. Grasp and control the guidewire where it protrudes from the hub. Hold the catheter near its tip and insert the tip through the skin. Then, stepwise, advance the entire length of the subclavian catheter in increments of several centimetres

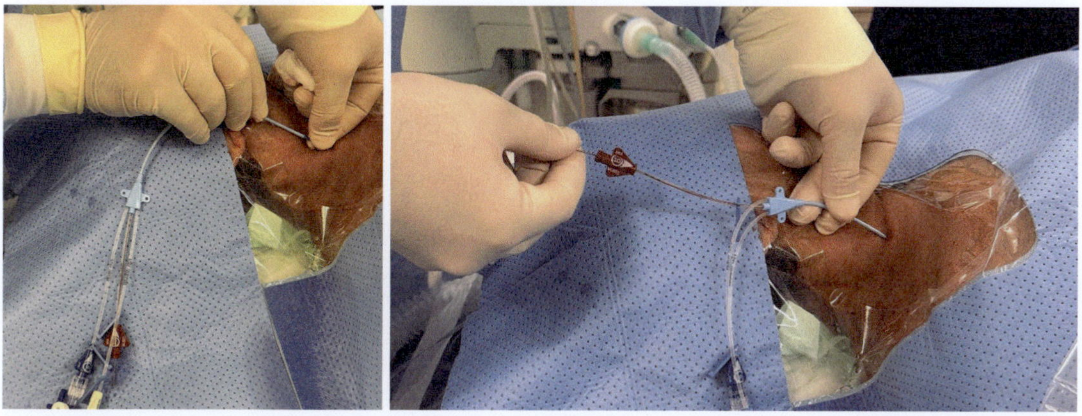

Fig. 4.13 Insert the central line over the wire

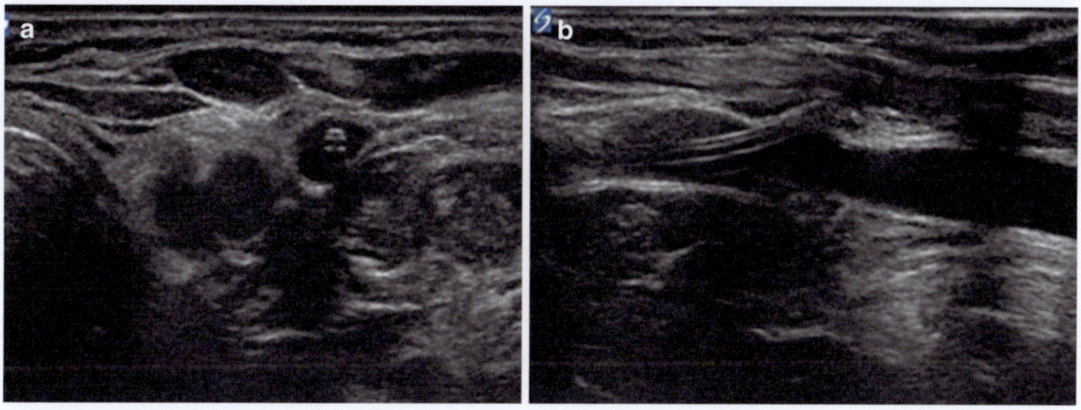

Fig. 4.14 Confirm catheter position in the vein: (**a**) short-axis view; (**b**) long-axis view

using a corkscrew motion as necessary. If ectopic heartbeats occur, slowly withdraw the catheter until the ectopy stops. Withdraw the guidewire while securely holding the catheter at the skin surface (Figs. 4.13 and 4.14).

After removing the wire, draw any air from the line and confirm venous blood flow into the hub. Then, using a 10-mL syringe and no excessive force, push 10 mL of saline into the line to clear it. Apply appropriate caps to the central line ports, secure the central line per institutional guidelines, and apply a sterile dressing to cover the insertion site.

By sealing the exit site with cyanoacrylate, we can avoid local bleeding, extraluminal bacterial contamination, and the risk of dislocation by increasing the stability of the catheter inside the skin breach [17, 18].

Consider using subcutaneous anchorage for catheter securement. This strategy could be safer and more effective than stabilisation, with skin-adhesive suture devices specially in high-risk patients for catheter dislodging (non-collaborative patients, diaphoresis, etc.) [19, 20].

A sterile dressing should be applied after completion of the procedure. Transparent, semi-permeable dressings have become a standard means of dressing catheter insertion sites, allowing visual inspection of the insertion site. Introducing an integrated gel pad containing a 2% concentration—by weight—of chlorhexidine gluconate into the transparent dressing should reduce skin and catheter colonisation. This will suppress the regrowth of microorganisms commonly related to catheter-related bloodstream infections at the catheter insertion site (Fig. 4.15).

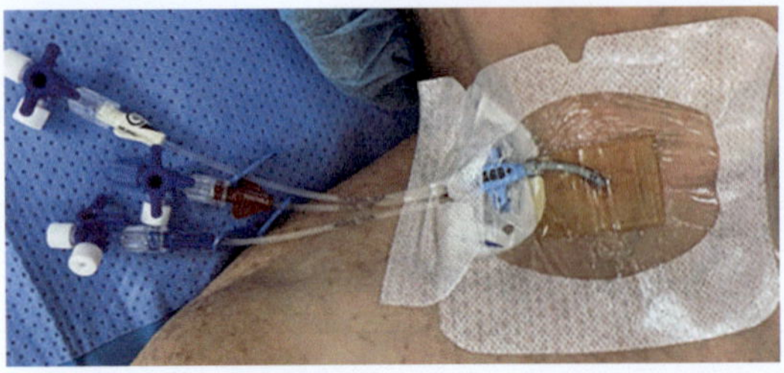

Fig. 4.15 Apply appropriate caps to the central line ports and secure the central line per institutional guidelines

Central Line Access Sites

Central venous catheters are commonly placed in veins in the neck (internal jugular vein), chest (subclavian vein or axillary vein), or groin (femoral vein). Additionally, for mid-term and long-term central venous access, the basilic and brachial veins are utilised for peripherally inserted central catheters (PICCs) [21].

Subclavian Approach

In the normal variant of human anatomy, each subclavian vein, the left and right, is a continuation of the axillary vein. The axillary vein begins at the lower border of the teres major and continues proximally until the lateral margin of the first rib, where it becomes the subclavian vein.

The subclavian vein site has the advantage of low rates of infectious and thrombotic complications. Additionally, it is accessible in trauma when a cervical collar negates the choice of the internal jugular vein. However, disadvantages include a higher relative risk of pneumothorax, less access to ultrasound for central venous catheter placement, and the non-compressible location posterior to the clavicle.

While ultrasound guidance methods have been documented and recommended, access at this site is often performed without ultrasound guidance using a landmark-guided technique.

Landmark Approach

For a long time, the anatomic landmark approach to subclavian cannulation was the standard of care and routine approach to this vessel. In recent years, the internal jugular and femoral veins have been more frequently accessed, largely due to the mandate to use ultrasonography for placement.

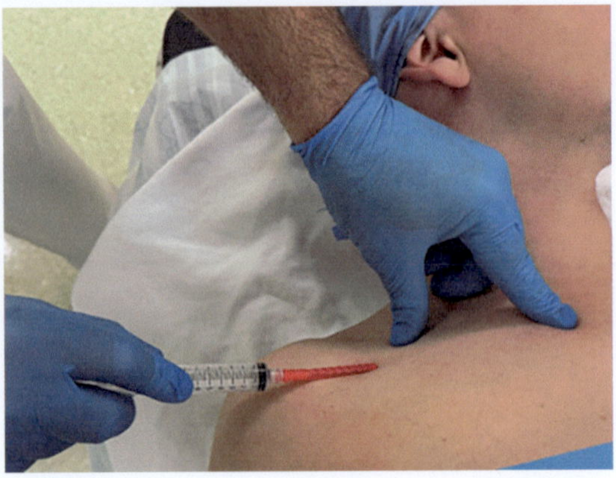

Fig. 4.16 Subclavian vein central line placement—landmark approach

If the right subclavian vein is selected, the left hand is used to palpate for external landmarks and vice versa for the left side. The index finger is placed in the sternal notch, and the thumb is at the clavicle's midpoint (Fig. 4.16).

The introducer needle is inserted immediately inferior to the clavicular midpoint at a shallow angle into the skin, aiming towards the sternal notch. It is important to guide the needle along a linear path and avoid a steep angle of the needle-related to the clavicle. Maintaining gentle negative pressure on the syringe plunger as you advance the needle is recommended. After a flash of blood appears in the barrel of the syringe, stop advancing. Sometimes, the proceduralist can feel the needle pop through the wall as it enters the lumen. Hold the syringe motionless in this spot. Even a slight movement may displace the needle tip from the vein (Fig. 4.16).

If no flash of blood appears in the syringe after 3–4 cm of insertion, withdraw the needle slowly. If the needle had initially entirely passed through the vein, a flash may now appear as you withdraw the needle tip back into the lumen. If a flash still does not appear, withdraw the needle almost to the skin surface, change direction, and try again to advance the needle into the vein. Do not change the direction of the needle while it is fully inserted.

Once the vein has been entered and venous blood is positively identified, proceed to place a catheter using the Seldinger technique.

Ultrasound Approach

The enhanced safety of ultrasound in the internal jugular position increases interest in ultrasound-guided cannulation of the subclavian vein as an alternative to the landmark approach. Evidence suggests that elective, real-time, ultrasound-guided cannulation of the subclavian vein may be more effective than the landmark-guided technique when performed by an experienced operator [7]. Compared with the landmark-guided technique, using ultrasound guidance for subclavian vein cannulation may reduce the rate of mechanical complications, decrease insertion time, and improve the overall success rate of the procedure [9, 22, 23].

The anatomical path below and behind the clavicle suggests that ultrasound may make the subclavian vein difficult to visualise. Moving the ultrasound probe laterally along the clavicle, however, enables visualisation of the infraclavicular proximal axillary vein and its surrounding structures and thus real-time ultrasound-guided needle advancement into, and cannulation of, the vein. Strictly speaking, while the technique is commonly referred to as "subclavian vein cannulation" in the published literature, anatomically, it is, in fact, an infraclavicular proximal axillary vein cannulation.

Ultrasound-guided subclavian vein cannulation can be performed using longitudinal (in-plane) and short (out-of-plane) axis views in the infraclavicular proximal axillary approach. In the short-axis view, the ultrasound beam is orientated in a transverse plane perpendicular to the target vessel, such that the vessel is seen as a circular structure. Advantages of this approach include better visualisation of nearby structures and relative ease for less experienced operators [14].

In contrast, the longitudinal axis approach is performed with the ultrasound beam aligned parallel to the target vessel, and the needle is maintained within the plane of the ultrasound beam. This approach's advantage is that the entire needle can be visualised as inserted into the vessel. A study comparing the longitudinal versus short-axis approach for subclavian vein catheterisation using simulation models demonstrated a decreased number of needle redirections and posterior wall punctures when using a longitudinal axis approach [24].

Short-axis view (out-of-plane) is obtained by placing the probe under and perpendicular to the clavicle at a point roughly delineating the lateral third of the clavicle with the orientation marker-directed cephalad. A transverse, or short-axis, image of the clavicle, subclavian vein, and subclavian artery should be visualised on the ultrasound screen. The vein and artery can be distinguished by assessing their compressibility or using colour-flow Doppler imaging to reveal pulsatility or non-pulsatility. The transducer should slowly move 1–2 cm towards the shoulder to obtain the best view of the subclavian vein. It is important to note that the lung lies inferior and posterior to the vessel; the pleura can be recognised as an echogenic linear structure below the subclavian vein.

First, obtain the short-axis view (in-plane) to gain the longitudinal axis view. Once the target vessel is identified, position it in the centre of the screen and rotate the transducer 90° to visualise the axillary vein/distal subclavian vein (Figs. 4.17 and 4.18).

After positioning the transducer so that the subclavian vein is near the centre of the ultrasound image, gently palpate the skin to confirm that the intended puncture site is aligned with the centre of the ultrasound transducer. The approximate depth of the subclavian vein and pleura can be determined using the depth marker located on the side of the ultrasound screen.

After aligning the introducer needle with the centre of the transducer, approach the site at an angle of 30–45°, with the long axis of the needle directed towards the sternal notch. Puncture the skin with the introducer needle at the centre of the transducer, being careful not to damage the sterile sheath. When the needle passes underneath the transducer, the needle tip and the tenting of soft tissue can be viewed on the ultrasound screen. As soon as the tip of the needle appears as a dot on the screen, be sure to keep the needle tip under direct ultrasound visualisation. The loca-

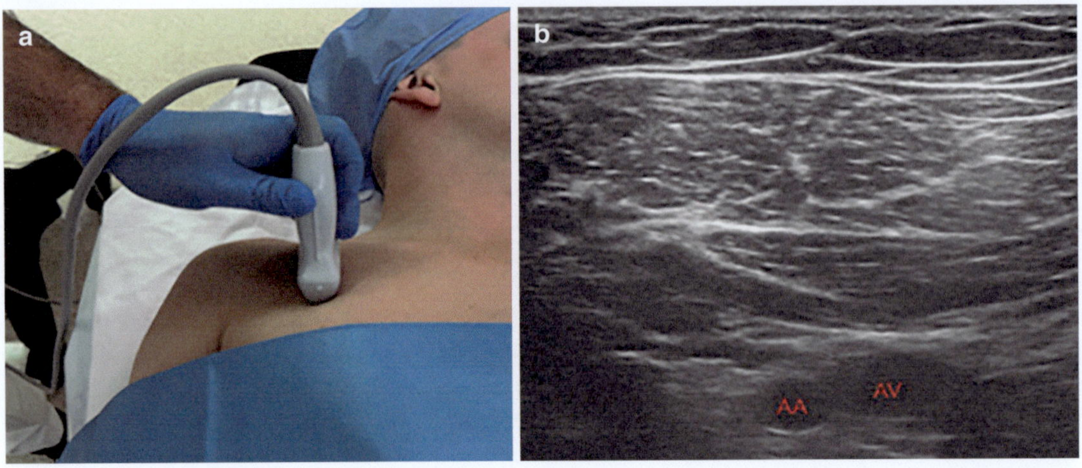

Fig. 4.17 A two-panel image. Panel (**a**) shows a medical professional using an ultrasound device on a patient's shoulder, with the patient lying down and covered with a blue drape. Panel (**b**) is an ultrasound image displaying internal structures with labels "AA" and "AV" indicating specific areas. The ultrasound image is in grayscale, showing various tissue layers

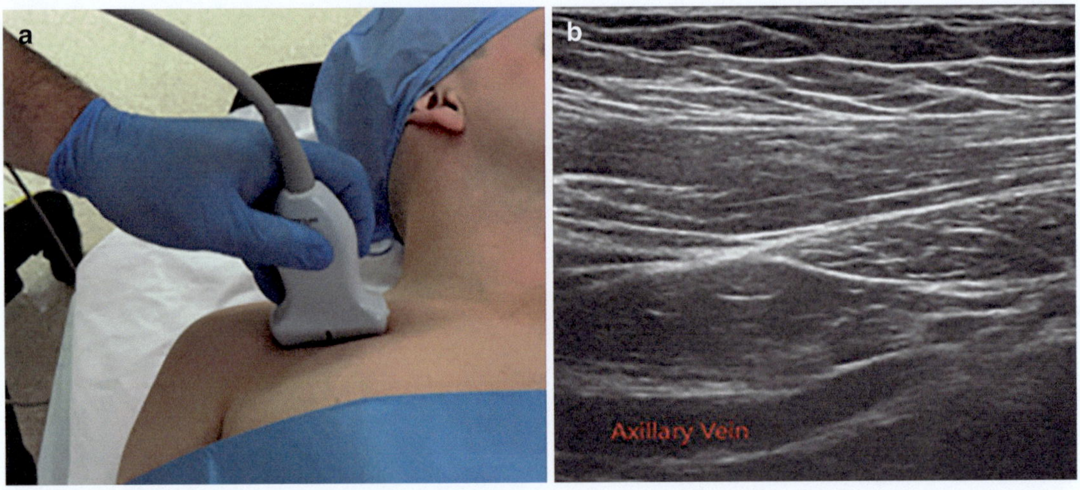

Fig. 4.18 A two-panel image showing a medical procedure and an ultrasound result. Panel (**a**) depicts a person lying down with a medical professional using an ultrasound probe on their shoulder area. The person is covered with a blue drape, and the professional is wearing blue gloves. Panel (**b**) displays an ultrasound image of the axillary region, with the text "Axillary Vein" in red, indicating the location of the vein

tion of the needle tip may also be visualised by tilting the transducer back and forth or by withdrawing the needle and realigning it. If the needle contacts the clavicle, withdraw the needle and use a slightly deeper trajectory. As you advance the needle towards the vein, maintain negative pressure in the syringe until the vein is punctured. Once the vein has been entered and venous blood is positively identified, place a catheter with the Seldinger technique.

To minimise the risk of a pneumothorax, always bear in mind the approximate depth of the subclavian vein and the extent to which the needle has been advanced.

Internal Jugular Vein

The internal jugular vein is often chosen for its reliable anatomy, accessibility, low complication rates, and ability to employ ultrasound guidance during the procedure. Its constant anatomic location makes it easier to catheterise than the subclavian vein.

The right internal jugular vein is usually preferred over the left for cannulation because it has a larger diameter and affords a straighter path to the superior vena cava and right atrium. It also avoids the higher left pleura and thoracic duct.

Traditionally, internal jugular vein cannulation has been performed using external anatomical landmarks and palpation to guide the needle's insertion into the vessel. However, this procedure may be difficult or unsuccessful depending on the operator's experience and the patient's anatomy.

Landmark Approach

The internal jugular vein is anterolateral to the common carotid artery, typically in the superior portion of the triangle created by the two heads of the sternocleidomastoid (SCM) muscle and the clavicle.

The carotid artery is usually palpated near the lateral side of the sternal head of the sternocleidomastoid, and the internal jugular vein usually lies superficial and lateral to the carotid artery. However, variant orientation of these vessels occurs regularly (Fig. 4.19). Age, gender, and side-related differences are present in the internal jugular vein—common carotid artery relationship and diameter. The orientation of the carotid artery and internal jugular vein to each other may also change if the position of the patient's head changes. Additionally, the anterior position of the internal jugular vein, relative to the common carotid artery, increases gradually with age [25]. Anatomical variations, such as duplications, fenestrations, agenesis, tributaries, and valves, may also lead to an increased failure rate and complications during the procedure, if unnoticed [26].

It is important to understand that the dynamics of the vessel can strongly correlate to respiratory and volumetric variations due to changes in intrathoracic pressures. The size of the veins varies with respiration (maximum diameter in patients not intubated occurs just before inspiration (before expiration in intubated patients)) and is increased by the Trendelenburg position, the Valsalva manoeuvre, humming, and external abdominal compression (Fig. 4.19) [27].

When anatomic landmarks are used, the internal jugular vein site can be accessed anteriorly, centrally, or posteriorly above the SCM bifurcation. The central approach to the internal jugular vein is most used, which may decrease the chance of pleural or carotid arterial puncture.

Gently palpate the carotid arterial pulse using three fingers to appreciate the artery's course and not to compress the adjacent internal jugular vein, considering that a compressed venous lumen is difficult to cannulate.

Insert procedural needles into the anterior cervical triangle's apical area, superior angle, just lateral to the carotid pulse, at a 30–40° angle into the skin, aiming towards the ipsilateral nipple.

Maintain carotid artery palpation during needle insertions, keeping the needle lateral to the artery to avoid impaling it. Once the vein has

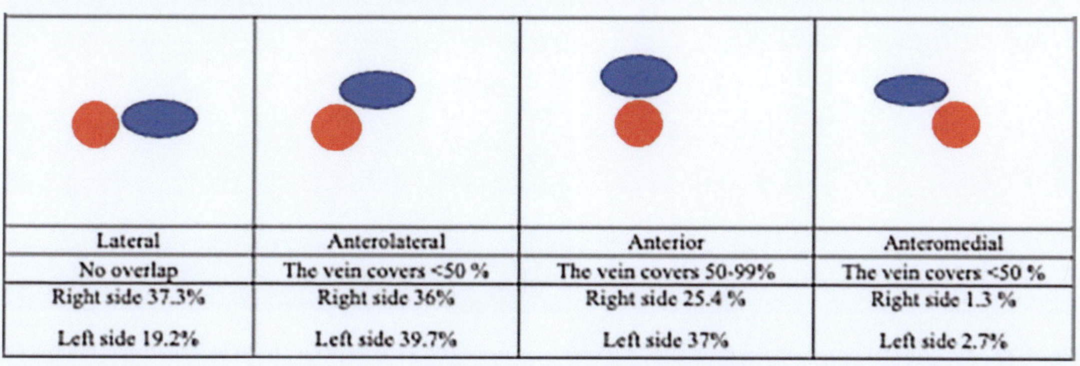

Lateral	Anterolateral	Anterior	Anteromedial
No overlap	The vein covers <50 %	The vein covers 50-99%	The vein covers <50 %
Right side 37.3%	Right side 36%	Right side 25.4 %	Right side 1.3 %
Left side 19.2%	Left side 39.7%	Left side 37%	Left side 2.7%

Fig. 4.19 Classification of the anatomical relationship between the internal jugular vein and common carotid artery

been entered and venous blood is positively identified, proceed to place a catheter with the Seldinger technique.

A micro-puncture needle is often used to find the internal jugular vein first (before inserting the larger introducer needle) so that if the needle aberrantly impales the carotid artery, less bleeding and hematoma result.

Ultrasound Approach

Variations in external landmarks and internal anatomy can make landmark-guided cannulation challenging. With ultrasound guidance for the placement of internal jugular lines, we can increase the likelihood of successful cannulation and reduce the risk of complications.

We may position the transducer to provide a cross-sectional or a longitudinal view. The large vessels and needle parallel the ultrasound beam in the longitudinal view. In this view, the entire shaft and tip of the needle and the course of a single vessel can be visualised. The anatomy and needle are perpendicular to the ultrasound beam in the transverse approach. Structures are visualised in cross-section, allowing us to identify both the internal jugular vein and the common carotid artery (Figs. 4.20 and 4.21).

Whichever view we select, we should attempt to locate the tip of the needle in relation to the ultrasound beam and the internal jugular vein. This is especially important when viewing the structures in cross-section since the needle will appear only as a dot on the screen, making it difficult to determine the exact location of the tip [28].

Position the transducer so that the resulting image on the screen correlates with the orientation of the anatomy. Place the probe parallel and cephalad to the clavicle along the sternocleidomastoid muscle.

The common carotid artery will be pulsating, making it difficult to compress. The internal jugular vein will be larger and non-pulsating, and it is easily compressed. Gently compress the internal jugular vein with the transducer to ensure that it is patent. Slight pressure is sufficient to collapse the lumen of the internal jugular vein.

We should attain an optimal cross-sectional image of the internal jugular vein using short-axis ultrasound guidance. Press lightly with the probe tip to avoid distorting the image size and shape of the vein. Slide the probe transversely as needed to place the imaged vein at the centre of the ultrasound screen. When the vein is centred on the ultrasound screen, the midpoint of the probe becomes a surface marker designating the luminal centre of the underlying vein.

When we have identified the entry site, insert the finder needle at a 45° angle to the skin, aiming towards the patient's ipsilateral nipple, with gentle suction applied to the syringe. Once the vein has been entered and venous blood is positively identified, place a catheter with the Seldinger technique.

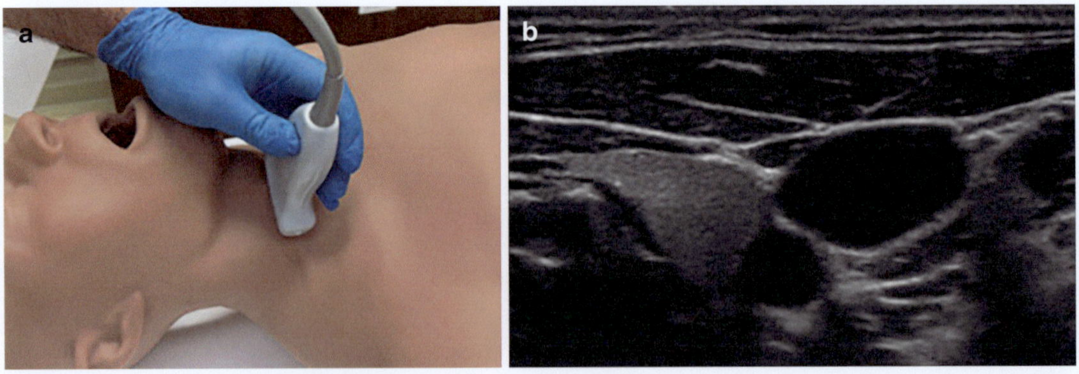

Fig. 4.20 A two-panel image. Panel (**a**) shows a person performing an ultrasound procedure on a mannequin's neck, using a handheld device. The person is wearing blue gloves. Panel (**b**) displays an ultrasound image of the neck area, showing various tissue layers and structures in grayscale

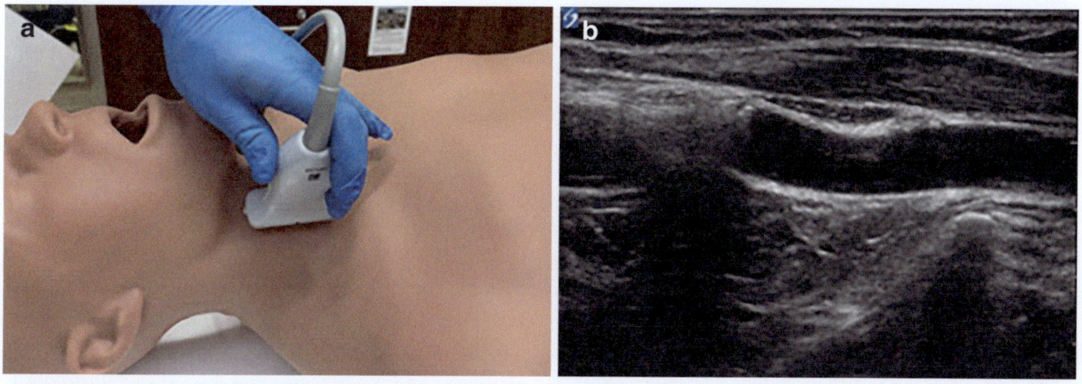

Fig. 4.21 A two-panel image showing an ultrasound procedure. Panel (**a**) depicts a person wearing blue gloves holding an ultrasound probe against the neck of a medical mannequin. Panel (**b**) displays the resulting ultrasound image, showing the internal structures of the neck with varying shades of gray. The image highlights the process and outcome of using ultrasound technology for medical examination

Femoral Vein

The femoral site is sometimes preferable in critically ill patients because the groin is free of other resuscitation equipment and devices, which may be required for monitoring and airway access. Central venous access in the common femoral vein offers the advantage of being an easily compressible site, which may be helpful in trauma and other coagulopathic patients. Additionally, unlike the internal jugular and subclavian sites, iatrogenic pneumothorax is not a concern. Patients may be more comfortable with a femoral CVC because it allows relatively free movement of the arms and legs compared to other sites. However, femoral CVCs are typically associated with increased thrombotic complications and likely an increased rate of catheter-associated infections. However, studies have shown conflicting results about the real risk of infection when the proper sterile technique is used [29–31].

The common femoral vein is the ideal to puncture when performing central venous access at the femoral site. The common femoral vein lies within the "femoral triangle" in the inguinal-femoral region. This region is bordered by the inguinal ligament superiorly, the adductor longus medially, and the sartorius muscle laterally. Within the femoral triangle, the common femoral vein is enclosed within the femoral sheath, which lies medial to the femoral artery. The common femoral vein receives several tributaries within this region, including the great saphenous and anterior saphenous veins. These veins can be inadvertently cannulated during the procedure and initially misinterpreted as femoral vein cannulation.

Landmark Approach

When obtaining central venous access in the femoral vein, the key anatomical landmarks to identify in the inguinal-femoral region are the inguinal ligament and the femoral artery pulsation. Using your index and middle fingers, locate the arterial pulsation along the inguinal ligament at the midpoint between the anterior superior iliac spine and the pubic symphysis. The insertion point of the femoral CVC is 1–2 cm inferior to the inguinal ligament and 1–2 cm medial to the maximal pulse of the femoral artery. Puncture the skin at a 30–45° angle to the skin (Fig. 4.22).

Ensure that the vein is punctured below the level of the inguinal ligament. A puncture above the inguinal ligament is, in fact, a puncture of the external iliac vein. The external iliac vein is a deep retroperitoneal structure. If it is lacerated and begins to bleed, it will be impossible to place pressure on the puncture wound.

Once the vein has been entered and venous blood is positively identified, proceed to place a catheter using the Seldinger technique.

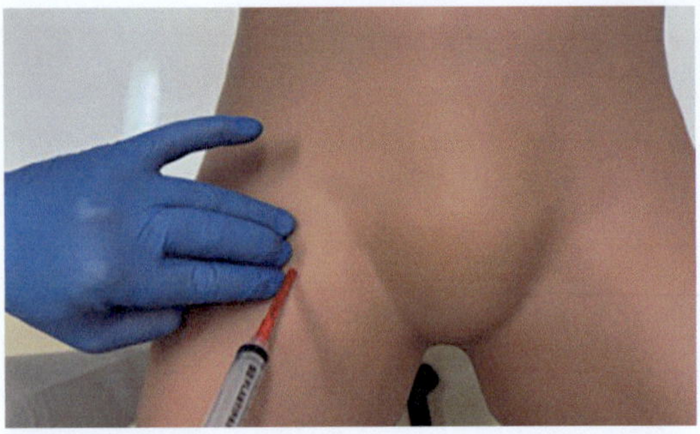

Fig. 4.22 Femoral vein central line placement—landmark approach

Ultrasound Approach

When we use ultrasound guidance for performing central venous access at the femoral site, we can assess the relationship of vessels to each other and other surrounding structures. We can also determine vessel depth, calibre, and patency. Venous thrombosis may appear as an echogenicity, grey irregularity, in the lumen but is often diagnosed because the thrombosed vein is incompressible. Thrombosis disqualifies the vein as a suitable cannulation site.

Using short-axis ultrasound guidance, attain an optimal cross-sectional image of the femoral vein 1–2 cm inferior to the inguinal ligament. Press lightly with the probe tip to avoid distorting the image size and shape of the vein. When the vein is centred on the ultrasound screen, the midpoint of the probe becomes a surface marker designating the luminal centre of the underlying vein. On the ultrasound screen, measure the depth to the centre of the vein. When using short-axis ultrasound guidance, insert procedural needles into the skin at a point distal and perpendicular to the midpoint of the probe, by the same distance as the vein depth. Then, initially advance the needle into the skin at a 45° angle directed towards the midpoint of the probe. Once the vein has been entered and venous blood is positively identified, proceed to place a catheter with the Seldinger technique (Fig. 4.23).

Peripherally Inserted Central Catheters

Peripherally inserted central catheters (PICCs) are a subset of central venous catheters. They are 50–60 cm long; single-, double-, or triple-lumen catheters are placed in a peripheral arm vein and terminated in the thorax. The length is necessary since it must reach from the area of the antecubital fossa to the superior vena cava. With an increasing need to use one catheter for multiple purposes, including injections for radiologic imaging, certain PICC types can accommodate power injections of up to 300 psi (pounds per square inch) at 5 mL/s [32]. The power injectable catheters need to be adequately labelled for this purpose. Most catheters are capable of withstanding up to 40 psi.

Peripherally inserted central catheters are placed through the basilic, brachial, cephalic, or, very rarely, medial cubital vein of the arm.

The basilic vein is chosen due to its larger size and superficial location. The basilic vein is usually accessed between the axilla and the antecubital fossa. Originating from the dorsal venous network of the hand, the basilic vein travels on the medial aspect of the upper extremity. After combining with the brachial vein, the axillary vein is formed, which becomes the subclavian vein at the border of the first rib and continues centrally to become the brachiocephalic (innominate) vein. The basilic vein has the straightest route to its destination, as it courses through the axillary vein. Other factors that have been thought to make the basilic vein the superior choice for PICC lines are that it has the least number of valves, better haemodilution capabilities, and a shallower insertion angle compared to other veins.

If the basilic vein is not accessible or occluded, accessing the right brachial vein may be attempted. However, it runs deeper than the basilic vein and is close to the brachial artery and median nerve.

The cephalic vein is another option for PICC line placement, but it is smaller than the basilic vein and can pass through the upper arm very torturously.

The median cubital vein is prominent in the antecubital fossa and courses directly to the basilic vein. However, given its location in the antecubital fossa, constant bending at the elbow increases the risk of complications, such as mechanical phlebitis.

Depending on the patient's clinical condition, available resources, and the healthcare profes-

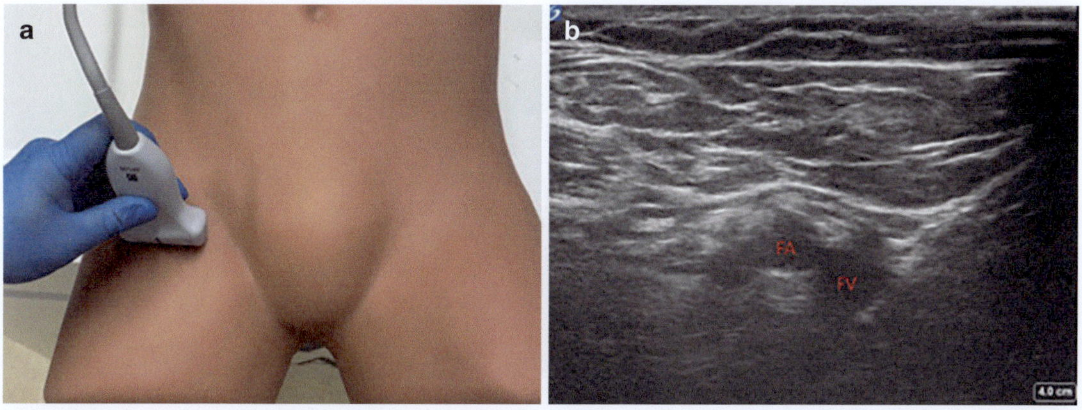

Fig. 4.23 A two-panel image showing a medical procedure and an ultrasound. Panel (**a**) depicts a person's lower abdomen with a gloved hand holding an ultrasound probe against the skin. Panel (**b**) displays an ultrasound image of the same area, showing internal structures with two red markers labeled "X" and "Y." The scale in the bottom right corner indicates 0.4 cm

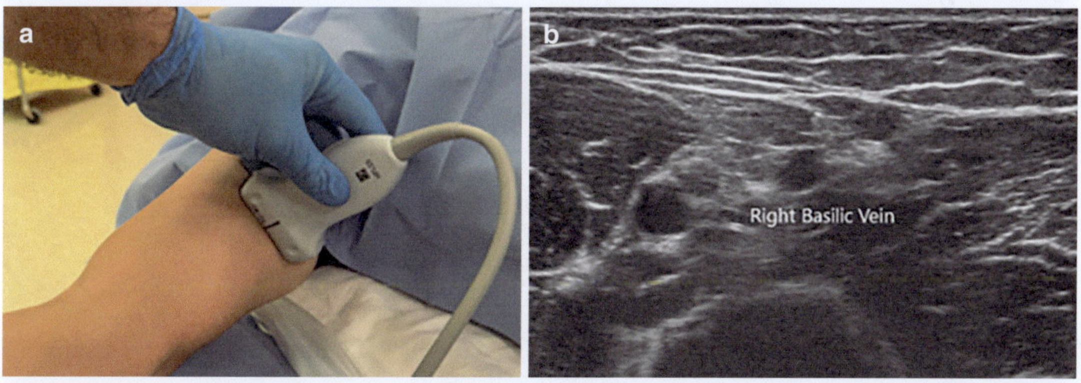

Fig. 4.24 A two-panel image showing an ultrasound procedure. Panel (**a**) depicts a person wearing blue gloves holding an ultrasound probe against a patient's arm, which is covered with a blue drape. Panel (**b**) displays an ultrasound image with the label "Right Basilic Vein," showing the vein's structure in grayscale

sional's preference, PICC line insertion can be performed at the bedside by several practitioners performing ultrasound-guided placement or a radiologist who may use fluoroscopic guidance to ensure intraoperative safety and correct catheter positioning.

Once the vein has been entered and venous blood is positively identified, proceed to place a catheter with the Seldinger technique. The Seldinger technique is the most commonly used method for placing PICCs. Peel-away cannulas or break-away needle methods are other options. However, they require large veins to accommodate larger-sized needles and introducers, which potentially exposes the patient to an increased risk of excessive bleeding.

Ultrasound-Guided Placement of a PICC

For ultrasound-guided placement, the arm should be at a 45–90° angle by the patient's side on an arm board, with the palm facing upward. The proceduralist needs to visualise the access vein with ultrasound directly. Anaesthetise the skin and subcutaneous tissue over the area of the vein with 1% lidocaine. Using the access needle, puncture the vein while directly visualising the needle tip. Ultrasound will confirm the correct positioning of the needle within the vein, as will blood return from the needle. An axial view of the vessel with the ultrasound will allow visualisation of the needle tip (Figs. 4.24 and 4.25).

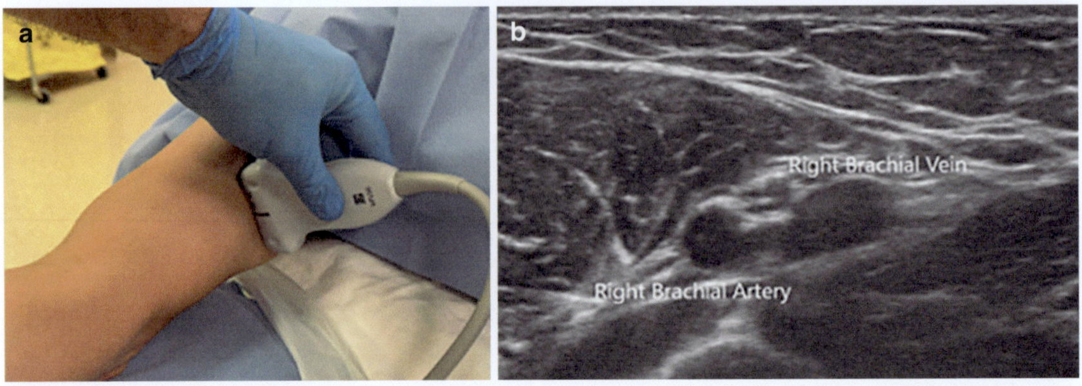

Fig. 4.25 A two-panel image showing a medical procedure and an ultrasound. Panel (**a**) depicts a person wearing blue gloves using an ultrasound probe on a patient's arm. Panel (**b**) is an ultrasound image showing the right brachial vein and right brachial artery, labeled in white text. The ultrasound displays the anatomical structures in grayscale

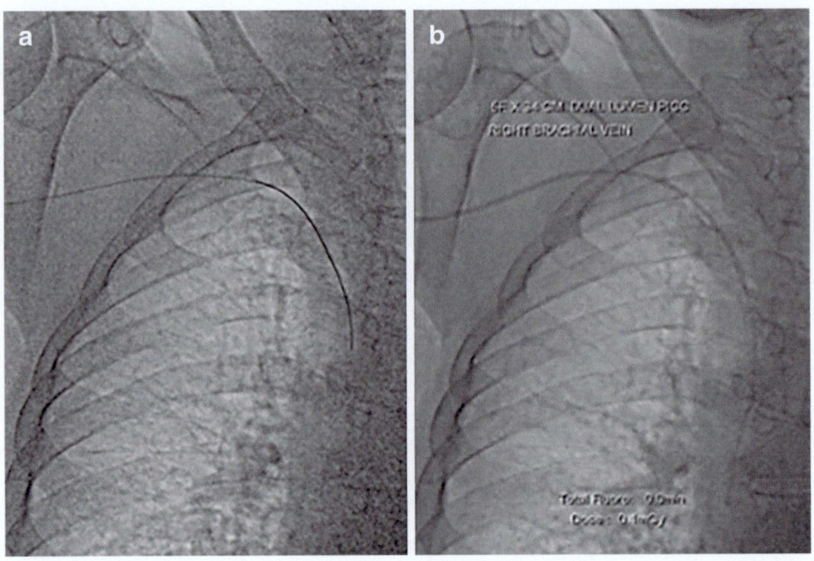

Fig. 4.26 The guidewire (**a**) and PICC catheter (**b**) position under fluoroscopic guidance

Fluoroscopically Guided Placement of a PICC

PICC line insertion under fluoroscopic guidance produces a continuous real-time X-ray image, allowing the clinician to ensure correct line placement. This technique works well for patients with small-diameter veins and unclear anatomy, reducing the risk of dangerous misplacement.

The procedure is similar to the ultrasound-guided placement, except that contrast material is inserted into the veins before the needle is placed. The guidewire is advanced under fluoroscopic guidance until the tip reaches the cavoatrial junction. The PICC catheter is threaded over the guidewire, ensuring the tip is positioned correctly under fluoroscopic guidance (Fig. 4.26) [33].

Post Central Venous Cannulation Assessment

Tip Placement Verification

Verifying the tip placement prevents potential complications from mechanical trauma of the catheter against the cardiac wall or infusion of fluids, medications, or nutrition into non-vasculature or inappropriate vasculature. Proper placement also decreases the incidence of dislodgment, vessel wall erosion and stenosis, and device dysfunction.

An assessment of tip position can be performed during or after the procedure. Ideally, tip position should be checked during the insertion by fluoroscopy, intracavity ECG, or ultrasound. Still, because the typical diagnostic tool used for this is chest radiography, the check is generally post-procedural.

Fluoroscopy is accurate but expensive; it may be logistically difficult or impossible, and it involves radiation exposure. Fluoroscopy can be used to verify tip placement if this method is being used to insert the catheter (Fig. 4.27).

Electrocardiogram-guided CVC placement is well tolerated and cost-effective, but it cannot be used when the P wave is not detectable, for example, in atrial arrhythmias. The electrocardiogram tip location allows the proceduralist to observe changes in the heart's electrical activity, focusing on the patient's P wave as the catheter tip advances through the superior vena cava, cavoatrial junction, and into the right atrium. This allows for accurate positioning of the catheter tip within the optimal range (Fig. 4.28) [34].

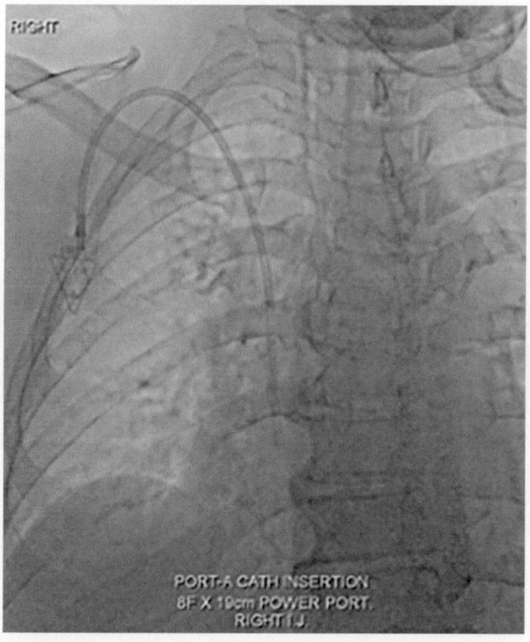

Fig. 4.27 Fluoroscopy after port catheter insertion

Ultrasound can be used as transthoracic echocardiography or trans-oesophageal echocardiography to confirm the tip position [35] directly. Transthoracic echocardiography may allow direct visualisation of the tip in the atrium and indirect visualisation at the cavoatrial junction [36]. It requires a particular ultrasound probe (convex phased array), specific training, and an echo-contrast medium. It may be difficult or impossible in obese patients after recent open-abdomen surgery or when the stomach or the colon is overinflated with gas. Trans-oesophageal echocardiography is the accurate method for CVC tip detection, but it is expensive, invasive, and not widely available (Fig. 4.29) [37].

Radiography has been the most frequently used method for tip confirmation but can present many challenges. Specific challenges include obtaining, interpreting, and reporting radiography [38, 39]. Furthermore, exposure to radiography emits harmful ionising radiation, which can increase the long-term risk of cancer. However, guidelines inform us that radiography should be justified, and the potential benefits of the exposure should outweigh the risks. If used, the chest radiograph is always obtained immediately after catheter insertion to rule out pneumothorax and document tip placement (Fig. 4.30).

Unlike subclavian and jugular venous catheters, femoral ones can be used immediately. Radiographic confirmation is not required if the catheter is operating correctly. A post-procedure abdominal film should be performed to confirm the catheter course and tip position if the catheter is not functioning correctly. Although it may be acceptable to have the catheter tip residing in the iliac vein for short-term use, the distal tip of femoral catheters should generally be located above the confluence of the iliac veins.

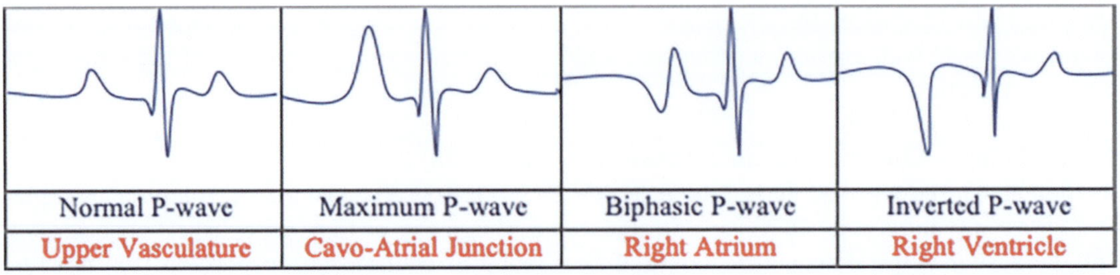

Fig. 4.28 Electrocardiogram-guided central venous catheter placement

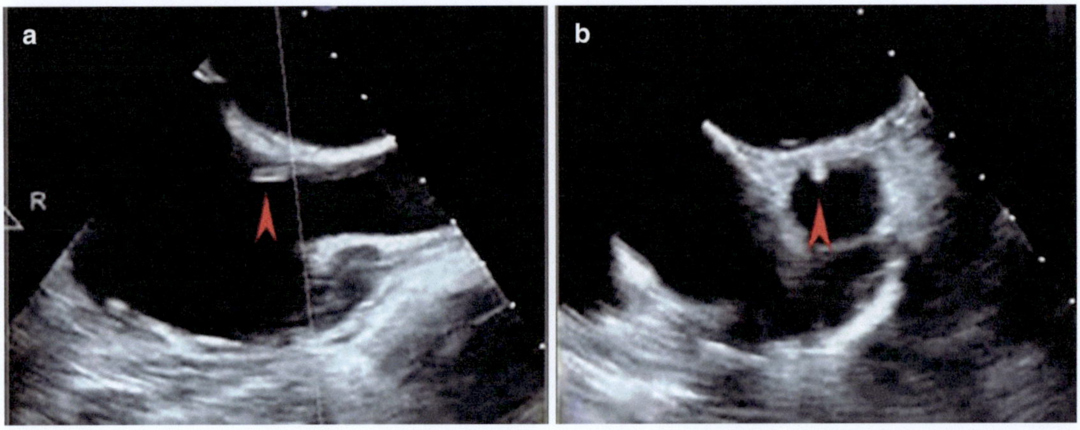

Fig. 4.29 Two-panel ultrasound images labeled "**a**" and "**b**" showing heart structures. Both panels feature a red arrow indicating specific areas of interest. The images display different cross-sectional views of the heart, highlighting anatomical features. The background is predominantly black, typical of ultrasound imaging

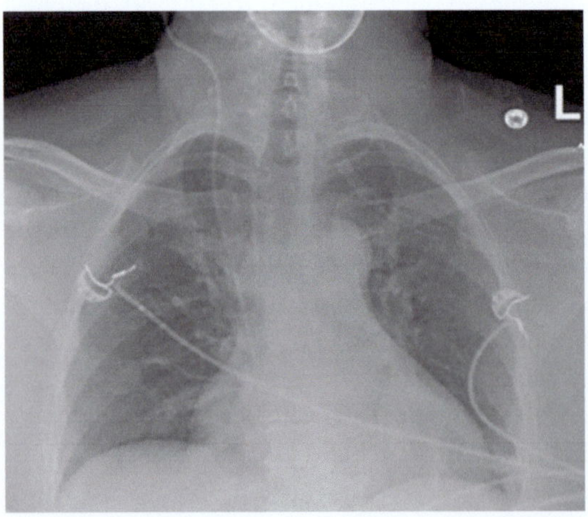

Fig. 4.30 Chest radiography of central venous catheter

Pearls and Highlights

When performed correctly, inserting a central venous catheter is safe, productive, and potentially life-saving. However, particular clinical pearls should be at the forefront of the proceduralist's mind when performing this procedure.

- Whenever possible, take the time to prepare for the procedure thoroughly, and ensure that all necessary personnel and equipment are in the room and readily available.
- Due to changes in intrathoracic pressures, vessel dynamics can strongly correlate with respiratory and volumetric variations. The size

of the veins varies with respiration and is increased by the Trendelenburg position, the Valsalva manoeuvre, and external abdominal compression.

- When access is performed with ultrasound, the internal jugular, subclavian, and femoral veins have higher success rates and fewer complications.
- Ensure that sterile products are not contaminated and that there is no evidence of damage to the packaging. Follow sterile procedures at all times.
- Never use excessive force during any part of this procedure.
- The proceduralist must always hold the guidewire inside the patient. Otherwise, the wire can be lost and migrate into the right ventricle or inferior vena cava, leading to additional invasive procedures to recover it.
- When using the internal jugular or subclavian site for access, obtain a stat portable chest X-ray immediately after line placement to ensure no pneumothorax and that the line terminates in the superior vena cava.
- The consistent use of transparent, semipermeable dressings ensures optimal protection and breathability of the exit site, additional stabilisation of the catheter, and reduction in the risk of skin-related injury.

References

1. Beheshti MV. A concise history of central venous access. Tech Vasc Interv Radiol. 2011;14(4):184–5. https://doi.org/10.1053/j.tvir.2011.05.002. PMID: 22099008.
2. Spencer TR, Pittiruti M. Rapid Central Vein Assessment (RaCeVA): a systematic, standardised approach for ultrasound assessment before central venous catheterisation. J Vasc Access. 2019;20(3):239–49. https://doi.org/10.1177/1129729818804718. Epub 2018 Oct 4. PMID: 30286688.
3. Brescia F, Pittiruti M, Ostroff M, Biasucci DG. Rapid Femoral Vein Assessment (RaFeVA): a systematic protocol for ultrasound evaluation of the veins of the lower limb to optimise the insertion of femorally inserted central catheters. J Vasc Access. 2021;22(6):863–72. https://doi.org/10.1177/1129729820965063.
4. Brescia F, Pittiruti M, Spencer TR, Dawson RB. The SIP protocol update: eight strategies, incorporating Rapid Peripheral Vein Assessment (RaPeVA), to minimise complications associated with peripherally inserted central catheter insertion. J Vasc Access. 2022;25:5–13. https://doi.org/10.1177/11297298221099838.
5. van de Weerdt EK, Biemond BJ, Baake B, Vermin B, Binnekade JM, van Lienden KP, Vlaar APJ. Central venous catheter placement in coagulopathic patients: risk factors and incidence of bleeding complications. Transfusion. 2017;57(10):2512–25. https://doi.org/10.1111/trf.14248. Epub 2017 Aug 30. PMID: 28856685.
6. Tercan F, Ozkan U, Oguzkurt L. US-guided placement of central vein catheters in patients with disorders of hemostasis. Eur J Radiol. 2008;65(2):253–6. https://doi.org/10.1016/j.ejrad.2007.04.002. Epub 2007 May 4. PMID: 17482407.
7. Schulman PM, Gerstein NS, Merkel MJ, Braner DA, Tegtmeyer K. Ultrasound-guided cannulation of the subclavian vein. N Engl J Med. 2018;379(1):e1. https://doi.org/10.1056/NEJMvcm1406114. PMID: 29972747.
8. Brass P, Hellmich M, Kolodziej L, Schick G, Smith AF. Ultrasound guidance versus anatomical landmarks for internal jugular vein catheterisation. Cochrane Database Syst Rev. 2015;1(1):CD006962. https://doi.org/10.1002/14651858.CD006962.pub2. PMID: 25575244; PMCID: PMC6517109.
9. Brass P, Hellmich M, Kolodziej L, Schick G, Smith AF. Ultrasound guidance versus anatomical landmarks for subclavian or femoral vein catheterization. Cochrane Database Syst Rev. 2015;1(1):CD011447. https://doi.org/10.1002/14651858.CD011447. PMID: 25575245; PMCID: PMC6516998.
10. Troianos CA, Hartman GS, Glas KE, Skubas NJ, Eberhardt RT, Walker JD, Reeves ST, Councils on Intraoperative Echocardiography and Vascular Ultrasound of the American Society of Echocardiography; Society of Cardiovascular Anesthesiologists. Special articles: guidelines for performing ultrasound guided vascular cannulation: recommendations of the American Society of Echocardiography and the Society of Cardiovascular Anesthesiologists. Anesth Analg. 2012;114(1):46–72. https://doi.org/10.1213/ANE.0b013e3182407cd8. Epub 2011 Nov 29. PMID: 22127816.
11. Bodenham Chair A, Babu S, Bennett J, Binks R, Fee P, Fox B, Johnston AJ, Klein AA, Langton JA, Mclure H, Tighe SQ. Association of Anaesthetists of Great Britain and Ireland: safe vascular access 2016. Anaesthesia. 2016;71(5):573–85. https://doi.org/10.1111/anae.13360. Epub 2016 Feb 17. Erratum in: Anaesthesia. 2016;71(12):1503. PMID: 26888253; PMCID: PMC5067617.
12. Lamperti M, Biasucci DG, Disma N, Pittiruti M, Breschan C, Vailati D, Subert M, Traškaitė V, Macas A, Estebe JP, Fuzier R, Boselli E, Hopkins P. European Society of Anaesthesiology guide-

lines on peri-operative use of ultrasound-guided for vascular access (PERSEUS vascular access). Eur J Anaesthesiol. 2020;37(5):344–76. https://doi.org/10.1097/EJA.0000000000001180.
13. Peters JL, Belsham PA, Garrett CP, et. al. Doppler ultrasound technique for safer percutaneous catheterization of the infraclavicular subclavian vein. Am J Surg. 1982;143:391–3.
14. Lamperti M, Bodenham AR, Pittiruti M, Blaivas M, Augoustides JG, Elbarbary M, Pirotte T, Karakitsos D, Ledonne J, Doniger S, Scoppettuolo G, Feller-Kopman D, Schummer W, Biffi R, Desruennes E, Melniker LA, Verghese ST. International evidence-based recommendations on ultrasound-guided vascular access. Intensive Care Med. 2012;38(7):1105–17. https://doi.org/10.1007/s00134-012-2597-x. Epub 2012 May 22. PMID: 22614241.
15. Saugel B, Scheeren TWL, Teboul JL. Ultrasound-guided central venous catheter placement: a structured review and recommendations for clinical practice. Crit Care. 2017;21:225. https://doi.org/10.1186/s13054-017-1814-y.
16. Seldinger SI. Catheter replacement of the needle in percutaneous arteriography. A new technique. Acta Radiol Suppl (Stockholm). 2008;434:47–52. https://doi.org/10.1080/02841850802133386. PMID: 19023715.
17. Scoppettuolo G, Annetta M, Marano C, et al. Cyanoacrylate glue prevents early bleeding of the exit site after CVC or PICC placement. Crit Care. 2013;17(Suppl 2):P174. https://doi.org/10.1186/cc12112.
18. Pittiruti M, Annetta MG, Marche B, D'Andrea V, Scoppettuolo G. Ten years of clinical experience with cyanoacrylate glue for venous access in a 1300-bed university hospital. Br J Nurs. 2022;31(8):S4–S13. https://doi.org/10.12968/bjon.2022.31.8.S4. PMID: 35439068.
19. Brescia F, Pittiruti M, Roveredo L, Zanier C, Morabito A, Santarossa E, Da Ros V, Montico M, Fabiani F. Subcutaneously anchored securement for peripherally inserted central catheters: immediate, early, and late complications. J Vasc Access. 2023;24(1):82–6. https://doi.org/10.1177/11297298211025430. Epub 2021 Jun 17. PMID: 34137321.
20. Pinelli F, Pittiruti M, Van Boxtel T, et al. GAVeCeLT-WoCoVA Consensus on subcutaneously anchored securement devices for the securement of venous catheters: current evidence and recommendations for future research. J Vasc Access. 2021;22(5):716–25. https://doi.org/10.1177/1129729820924568.
21. Kolikof J, Peterson K, Baker AM. Central venous catheter. [Updated 2023 Jul 26]. In: StatPearls [Internet]. Treasure Island: StatPearls Publishing; 2023. Available from: https://www.ncbi.nlm.nih.gov/books/NBK557798/.
22. Fragou M, Gravvanis A, Dimitriou V, Papalois A, Kouraklis G, Karabinis A, Saranteas T, Poularas J, Papanikolaou J, Davlouros P, Labropoulos N, Karakitsos D. Real-time ultrasound-guided subclavian vein cannulation versus the landmark method in critical care patients: a prospective randomized study. Crit Care Med. 2011;39(7):1607–12. https://doi.org/10.1097/CCM.0b013e318218a1ae. PMID: 21494105.
23. Lalu MM, Fayad A, Ahmed O, Bryson GL, Fergusson DA, Barron CC, Sullivan P, Thompson C, Canadian Perioperative Anesthesia Clinical Trials Group. Ultrasound-guided subclavian vein catheterization: a systematic review and meta-analysis. Crit Care Med. 2015;43(7):1498–507. https://doi.org/10.1097/CCM.0000000000000973. PMID: 25803646.
24. Vogel JA, Haukoos JS, Erickson CL, Liao MM, Theoret J, Sanz GE, Kendall J. Is long-axis view superior to short-axis view in ultrasound-guided central venous catheterization? Crit Care Med. 2015;43(4):832–9. https://doi.org/10.1097/CCM.0000000000000823. PMID: 25517477; PMCID: PMC4436655.
25. Umaña M, García A, Bustamante L, Castillo JL, Martínez JS. Variations in the anatomical relationship between the common carotid artery and the internal jugular vein: an ultrasonographic study. Colomb Med [Internet]. 2015 [cited 2024 Jan 21];46(2):54–59. Available from: http://www.scielo.org.co/scielo.php?script=sci_arttext&pid=S1657-95342015000200002&lng=en.
26. Kosnik N, Kowalski T, Lorenz L, Valacer M, Sakthi-Velavan S. Anatomical review of internal jugular vein cannulation. Folia Morphol (Warsz). 2023;83:1. https://doi.org/10.5603/FM.a2023.0008. Epub ahead of print. PMID: 36794685.
27. Tufegdzic B, Khozenko A, Lee St John T, Spencer TR, Lamperti M. Dynamic variation of the axillary veins due to intrathoracic pressure changes: a prospective sonographic study. J Vasc Access. 2020;21(1):66–72. https://doi.org/10.1177/1129729819852204. Epub 2019 Jun 16. PMID: 31204560.
28. Ortega R, Song M, Hansen CJ, Barash P. Videos in clinical medicine. Ultrasound-guided internal jugular vein cannulation. N Engl J Med. 2010;362(16):e57. https://doi.org/10.1056/NEJMvcm0810156. PMID: 20410510.
29. American Society of Anesthesiologists Task Force on Central Venous Access, Rupp SM, Apfelbaum JL, Blitt C, Caplan RA, Connis RT, Domino KB, Fleisher LA, Grant S, Mark JB, Morray JP, Nickinovich DG, Tung A. Practice guidelines for central venous access: a report by the American Society of Anesthesiologists Task Force on Central Venous Access. Anesthesiology. 2012;116(3):539–73. https://doi.org/10.1097/ALN.0b013e31823c9569. PMID: 22307320.
30. Marik PE, Flemmer M, Harrison W. The risk of catheter-related bloodstream infection with femoral venous catheters as compared to subclavian and internal jugular venous catheters: a systematic review of the literature and meta-analysis. Crit Care Med. 2012;40(8):2479–85. https://doi.org/10.1097/CCM.0b013e318255d9bc. PMID: 22809915.

31. Arvaniti K, Lathyris D, Blot S, Apostolidou-Kiouti F, Koulenti D, Haidich AB. Cumulative evidence of randomized controlled and observational studies on catheter-related infection risk of central venous catheter insertion site in ICU patients: a pairwise and network meta-analysis. Crit Care Med. 2017;45(4):e437–48. https://doi.org/10.1097/CCM.0000000000002092. PMID: 27632678.
32. Hadaway L, Richardson D. Needleless connectors: a primer on terminology. J Infus Nurs. 2010;33(1):22–31. https://doi.org/10.1097/NAN.0b013e3181c65cc9. PMID: 20075681.
33. Montanarella MJ, Agarwal A, Moon B. Peripherally Inserted Central Catheter (PICC) line placement. [Updated 2024 Jan 10]. In: StatPearls [Internet]. Treasure Island: StatPearls Publishing; 2024. Available from: https://www.ncbi.nlm.nih.gov/books/NBK573064/.
34. Gullo G, Qanadli SD. ECG-based techniques to optimize peripherally inserted central catheters: rationale for tip positioning and practical use. Front Cardiovasc Med. 2022;9:765935. https://doi.org/10.3389/fcvm.2022.765935. PMID: 35600463; PMCID: PMC9120917.
35. Lamperti M, Pittiruti M. Central venous catheter tip position: another point of view. Eur J Anaesthesiol. 2015;32(1):3–4. https://doi.org/10.1097/EJA.0000000000000050.
36. Vezzani A, Brusasco C, Palermo S, Launo C, Mergoni M, Corradi F. Ultrasound localization of central vein catheter and detection of postprocedural pneumothorax: an alternative to chest radiography. Crit Care Med. 2010;38(2):533–8. https://doi.org/10.1097/CCM.0b013e3181c0328f. PMID: 19829102.
37. Ender J, Erdoes G, Krohmer E, Olthoff D, Mukherjee C. Transesophageal echocardiography for verification of the position of the electrocardiographically-placed central venous catheter. J Cardiothorac Vasc Anesth. 2009;23(4):457–61. https://doi.org/10.1053/j.jvca.2008.12.003. Epub 2009 Feb 13. PMID: 19217801.
38. Gefter WB, Hatabu H. Reducing errors resulting from commonly missed chest radiography findings. Chest. 2023;163(3):634–49. https://doi.org/10.1016/j.chest.2022.12.003. Epub 2022 Dec 10. PMID: 36513187.
39. Hsu JH, Wang CK, Chu KS, Cheng KI, Chuang HY, Jaw TS, Wu JR. Comparison of radiographic landmarks and the echocardiographic SVC/RA junction in the positioning of long-term central venous catheters. Acta Anaesthesiol Scand. 2006;50(6):731–5. https://doi.org/10.1111/j.1399-6576.2006.01025.x. PMID: 16987369.

Central Venous Catheter (CVC) Insertion Techniques

5

Insertion Techniques for Central Venous Catheters and Management of Catheter-Related Complications

Ilaria Donati

Modern central venous catheter (CVC) insertion techniques almost exclusively involve the use of ultrasound for vessel retrieval, visualization, and subsequent cannulation.

The central venous catheter began its history with the method of surgical exposure of the vessel, which was subsequently cannulated "on sight."

At the beginning of 90s, skin landmarks were identified that defined the point, more or less exactly, where to puncture with blind technique to cannulate the vessel.

This technique exposed the patient to numerous complications, some of which also greatly impacted the patient's health. Some of the most common include failure (even in experienced hands), arterial puncture, and the possibility of procuring pneumothorax, particularly with subclavian vein and internal jugular vein puncture.

To obviate these problems and simplify the life of the operators, attempts have gradually been made to improve performance with the use at first of Doppler technique and later, in the early years of our century with the use, increasingly widespread, of ultrasound.

The technique of finding the venous vessel with ultrasound requires a relatively fast learning curve and almost totally negates the possibility of failure.

It also allows one to be able to measure the caliber of the vessel to be cannulated and choose the best vessel for the patient's needs.

In accordance with the GAVeCeLT and SIAARTI guidelines, placement will be echo-guided (the use of ultrasound in the context of vascular access is considered to be performed with a 5–15 MHz linear probe in B Mode) after evaluation of the vascular heritage to determine the optimal venipuncture site by assessing caliber and collapsibility, depth, patency, and anatomical relationships with sensitive structures (arteries, nerves, pleura, trachea).

The external caliber of the catheter should never exceed one-third of the diameter of the vessel that receives it: this is in order to reduce a much-feared late complication that is vessel thrombosis.

It also cuts down the complications that were more frequent with the blind technique, namely, arterial puncture and pleural puncture.

This is allowed because with ultrasound, all structures adjacent to the target are easily detected allowing the operator to be precise in venipuncture.

I. Donati (✉)
Anesthesia Section Hospitals Area Sud,
Ausl Modena, Modena, Italy

R. Lanocita, M. Lamperti (eds.), *Practical Guide to Central Venous Cannulation*,
https://doi.org/10.1007/978-3-031-90326-7_5

How Do We Proceed Practically?

The purpose of this manual is to provide users with practical guidance that may be useful to them in their daily clinical practice.

For this reason, we will give a very practical and somewhat schematic outline of how to proceed for a central venous cannulation.

We will skip the phase of patient preparation and sterile field setup because it is the subject of previous chapters in this manual.

Choice of Venous Vessel and Its Measurement

When having to choose a central venous vessel for cannulation, several variables must be taken into consideration: patient's venous heritage; need for a long-term, medium-term, and short-term device: in case of a long-term catheter, we refer to the specific chapter in this manual.

For other time-related indications, the most indicated vessels are generally the internal jugular vein, the axillary vein bordering the subclavian, and, in special cases, the femoral vein.

In recent years, peripherally inserted central venous catheters (PICCs) have also come into use.

However, all cannulation sites involve the same technique.

- Careful excursus of the patient's venous supply with ultrasonography to assess the most appropriate vessel for the different circumstances: right/left internal jugular vein, right/left axillary vein, right/left femoral vein, right/left brachial vein, basilar vein, and right/left cephalic vein
- Ultrasonographic measurement of vessel caliber (expressed in millimeter) and subsequent choice of catheter caliber (expressed in French), which should be a maximum of one-third of the diameter of the vessel receiving it (Fig. 5.1)

The conversion factor between the two units of measurement is 1/3, i.e., 1 fr = 0.33 mm.

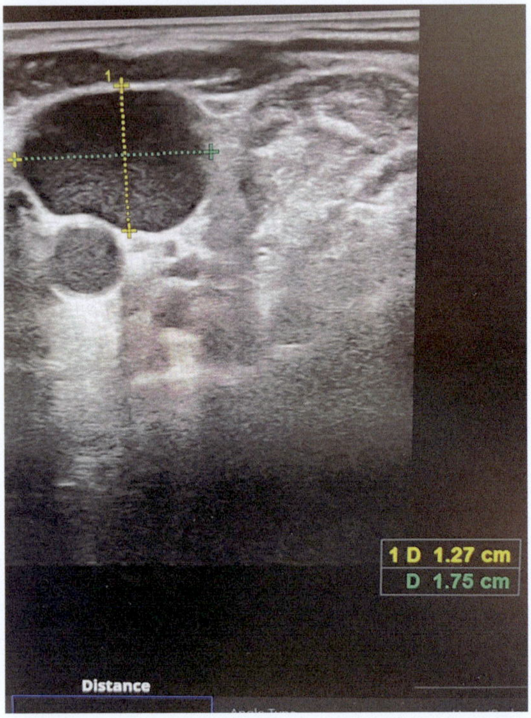

Fig. 5.1 Ultrasound measurement of vessel diameter

This greatly simplifies the choice of catheter gauge.

A vessel that measures 5 mm can accommodate a 5 fr catheter; one that measures 6 mm is a 6 fr catheter and so on.

Cannulation Technique

- The operator must use all the PPE and techniques necessary to perform a maneuver in complete sterility.
- Sterile field setup, preferably with 2% chlorhexidine in 70% alcohol solution. This choice prefers chlorhexidine to povidone iodine. In fact, chlorhexidine promotes almost instantaneous evaporation of the disinfectant, which is described as the best surgical disinfectant.
- Use for echo-guided venipuncture of micropuncture technique. Micropuncture technique refers to the use of needles and introducers with a maximum gauge of 21G. This is for the purpose of minimizing vessel wall trauma to reduce the risk of thrombosis, which is already

amplified by the presence of foreign body. In fact, we know that the main cause of vascular thrombosis is precisely to be found in wall damage. Minimizing wall damage therefore reduces the risk of thrombosis.

- Minimize the number of venipuncture attempts by using the ultrasound technique with in-plane view of the needle. The in-plain view allows visualization of the needle throughout its course from the skin, through the subcutaneous tissues to the vessel puncture. This also reduces complications such as arterial puncture and/or pleural puncture (in neck vessels).
- Technique with metal guide inside the needle (Seldinger)to slide the catheter into the vessel (with or without dilator-introducer peel-away complex).
- Attachment of the garrison to the skin using a sutureless technique, which decreases the risk of infection of the CVC emergence site.

Checking the Correct Positioning of the Catheter Tip

Proper placement of the CVC tip is critical to reduce the risk of one of the most feared complications, along with catheter-related infection, which is thrombosis of the vessel that houses the catheter. This complication carries high health risks for the CVC-carrying patient both because thrombosis can result in an embolism and because resolving it requires coagulating the patient with high-dose EBPM or even continuous infusion heparin before removing the device. These therapies expose the patient to risk of digestive or cerebral hemorrhage.

For all these reasons, placing the tip of the CVC correctly appears critical.

The best place to place the CVC tip is the transition between the right atrium and superior vena cava corresponding to the sinus node (Fig. 5.2).

Why there?

Typically, CVCs are placed for specific needs, such as high osmolarity therapy, administration

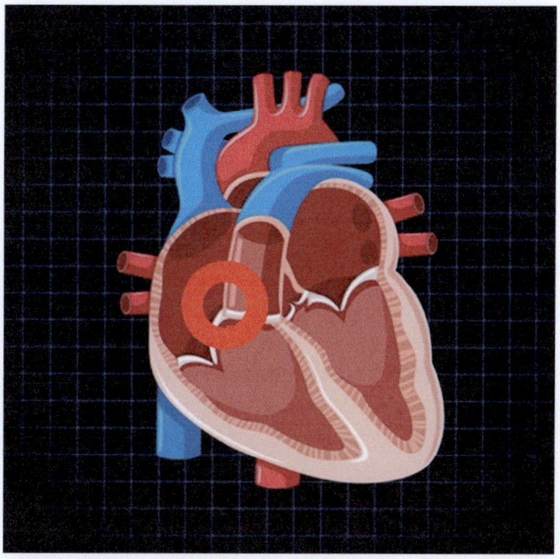

Fig. 5.2 The circle indicates the position of the sinus node. (Image courtesy of it.freepik.com/)

of urticant/vesicant drugs, and/or for PVC (central venous pressure) detection. Its misplacement could prove dangerous or provide incorrect monitoring indications.

Seeking a position of the tip in a large-caliber vessel, such as central vessels, is not sufficient to avoid complications.

We should try to place the tip in the place with the greatest laminar flow with the intention of minimizing the risk of foreign body thrombosis. In fact, with laminar blood flow, we avoid initiating the coagulation process that always starts with platelet adhesion.

Along the entire course of the superior vena cava, the flow is laminar, but placing the CVC further upstream would expose the catheter to risk of tip migration, for example, into contralateral subclavian or jugular vein, even for moderate efforts such as coughing or use of the abdominal press.

Placing the catheter further downstream (toward the right atrium) would expose the patient to arrhythmias and valvular injury, not to mention that in the atrial cavity, the blood flow becomes turbulent, thus increasing the thrombotic risk.

For all these reasons, detection of the catheter tip position appears crucial.

Central Venous Catheter Tip Detection Techniques

Over the years, numerous methods have been investigated to control the position of the tip of the implanted device.

Postprocedural control methods and intraprocedural methods have been developed.

Postprocedural Checkup with Chest X-Ray

Initially, control was exclusively radiographic.

This method, accurate enough when used by experienced operators, nevertheless suffers from being operator dependent. Not only by the operator who "reads" the radiographic image, but also by the operator (radiology technician) who performs the acquisition. Imperfect alignment between the X-ray machine and the patient can change the projection and distort the reading. Acquiring the image with patient in inspiratory or expiratory phase changes the relationships between the ribs, diaphragm, and bronchial tree. In principle, the catheter tip should be one space below the bronchial bifurcation (Fig. 5.3).

In addition, this method assesses the position of the tip after placement with the risk in case of imperfect placement of having to repeat the maneuver or otherwise act on the patient again to improve performance.

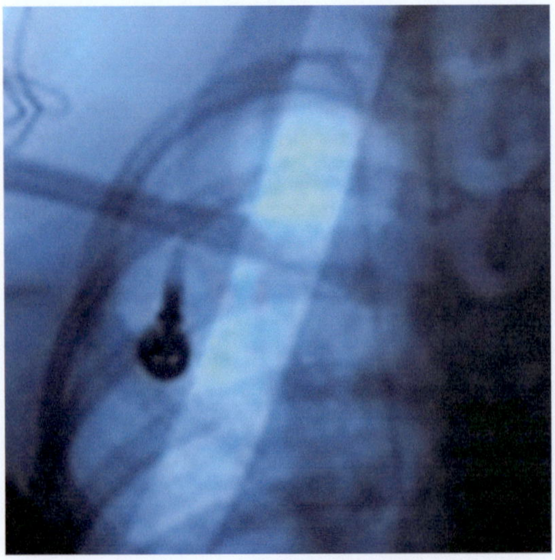

Fig. 5.3 Radiographic view of implanted Port

Intraprocedural Control with Brightness Amplifier (Fluoroscopy)

Checking the tip position with a luminance amplifier is superimposable to checking with postoperative radiography. The advantage is not having to repeat the maneuver but being able to apply the necessary corrections during the maneuver. The disadvantage is that the operator is exposed to irradiation along with the patient. In addition, not all environments are architecturally suitable for the use of radiation: in fact, environments with leaded walls are needed. Not least is the possibility of having a dedicated operator available to handle and use the brilliance amplifier. The image returned by the fluoroscope is superimposable to that of chest Rx. The main difference between the two methods lies in the fact that the chest X-ray provides a static and a posteriori image, whereas the fluoroscope has a dynamic and intraprocedural value.

Intraprocedural Check with Transesophageal Ultrasonography

Transesophageal ultrasonography is certainly a very appealing method of detecting the position of the catheter tip. Certainly not simple. A long learning curve is needed. As is well known, ultrasound does not allow echoes to pass through the bone and sends back a black image below which no structure can be detected. An attempt has been made to overcome this problem by using an ultrasound contrast agent (sulfur hexafluoride) that gives greater echogenicity to the blood flow. Injecting this contrast medium through the CVC allows for ultrasound evaluation of the flow and therefore localization of the tip. The method is quite investigative and not very precise.

This method requires personnel experienced in using the instrument (transesophageal ultrasound) generally reserved for cardiologists or cardiac anesthesiologists.

In addition, at the very least, more or less deep sedation is required for the patient undergoing the investigation.

All these reasons advise against, at least routinely, the use of this method, which is, moreover, very accurate and precise.

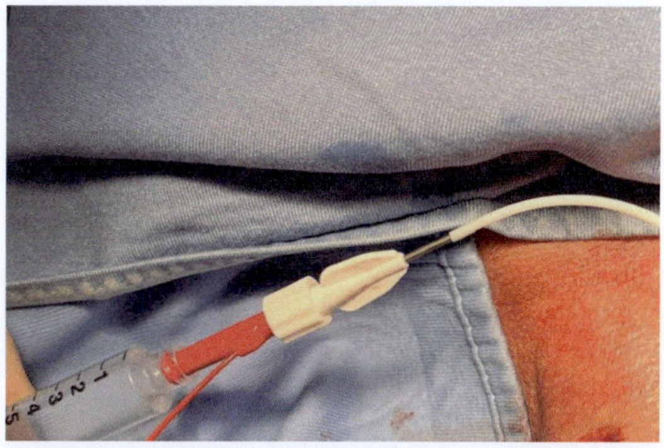

Fig. 5.4 Connection between "red" electrode and catheter

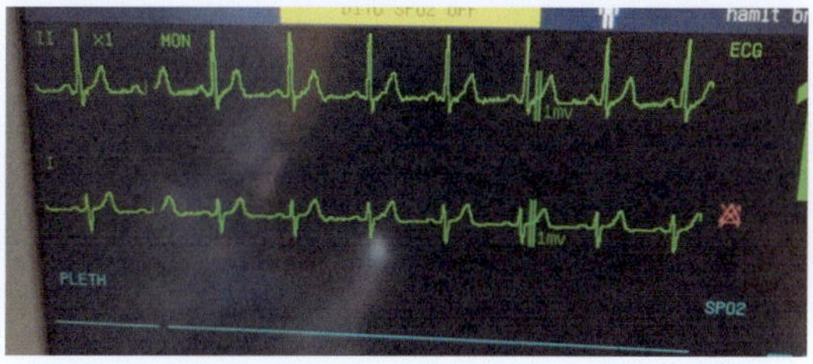

Fig. 5.5 P wave of normal ECG

Intraprocedural Control by Electrocardiographic Method

The electrocardiographic or endocavitary electrode method is a catheter tip localization system dating back to the 1980s, which fell into disuse for more than two decades and has recently seen a resurgence due to its simplicity of detection, short learning curve, and cost containment.

Costs are low compared with using the RX system to check the correct positioning of the catheter tip with savings also in radiation for the patient, the operator, and even the environment.

The electrocardiographic method has also evolved over time due to the interest of industry, which has put on the market several systems aimed at making the task easier for the operator by trying to make it even easier to place the catheter tip in the right place.

We will make a brief list of systems using the endocavitary electrode method.

Classical Endocavitary Electrode Method

This involves connecting a surface electrode (usually the "red" electrode) of the right arm to a column of water with electrolytes (0.9% NaCl solution) in turn connected to the catheter in place (Fig. 5.4).

In this way, the trace detectable at the monitor (in II lead) will be the one detected at the catheter tip.

The method takes advantage of the fact that anatomically at the transition between the superior vena cava and the right atrium, the perfect point for housing the catheter tip is the sinus node (natural and physiological pacemaker).

Electrocardiographically, it results in the transcription of the "P" wave of the ECG tracing (Fig. 5.5).

By reading the tracing with the endocavitary electrode, the shape of the P wave changes, and in particular, it is amplified the closer the tip is to the sinus node.

Advancing with the CVC until the maximum amplitude of the P wave is obtained undoubtedly tells us the correct position of the catheter tip (Fig. 5.6).

However, care should be taken that the P wave does not become negative with respect to the isoelectric line of the ECG.

This certainly indicates that the catheter tip has passed beyond the sinus node, the reading being a vector type reading (Fig. 5.7).

The method just described is simple to apply, has very low costs, does not involve a particularly long or demanding learning curve, is easily reproducible, and, with a printout of the two

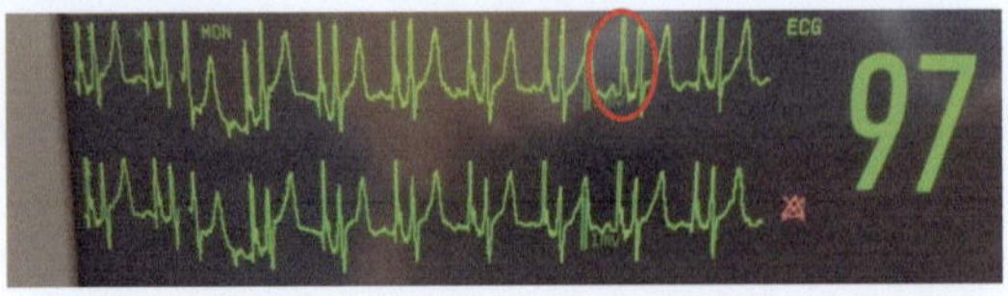

Fig. 5.6 Maximum P wave

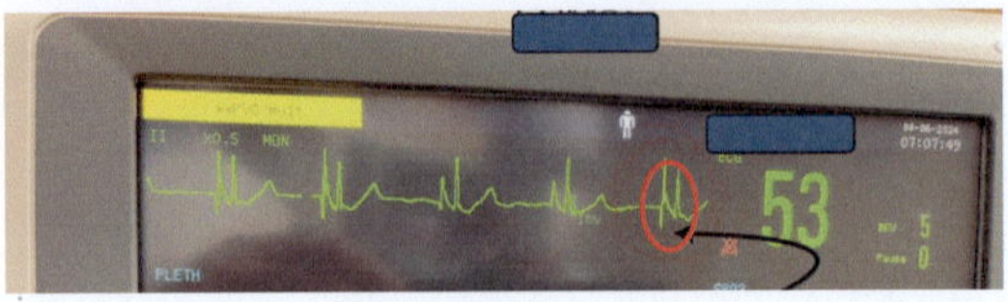

Fig. 5.7 Negative P wave

traces, external/endocavitary, also allows official documentation of correct placement.

The disadvantage of this method is that it is not applicable in the case of cardiac arrhythmias, particularly in the case of atrial fibrillation, the P wave reading being fundamental to the technique.

The electromedical industry provides some tools for tip localization with intraprocedural techniques. The basic principle on which they are based is the same as the intracavitary electrode technique (electrocardiographic method). These instruments have the advantage that they can also be used in cases of atrial arrhythmias, thanks to software that can "clean" the ECG trace of the abnormalities generated by the arrhythmia.

The two most widely used systems are PILOT® and SHERLOCK®.

We briefly expound the peculiarities of the two systems.

PILOT®

The main feature of this system is that it simultaneously acquires the intracavitary signal and the surface ECG in II lead to ensure an accurate comparison between the two waveforms.

Thanks to a specific algorithm, PILOT can automatically recognize and highlight the P wave facilitating the interpretation of the trace by the operator.

In addition, the system is able to assign a numerical value representing the amplitude of the P wave facilitating the recognition of the maximum value.

Improved over the intracavitary ECG method described above is the ability to also apply the ECG technique to patients with atrial fibrillation, a condition that has historically been a limitation to the applicability of this technique.

The system also provides a "Tip navigation" signal (Piloting® mode). Through this function, it is possible to determine from the earliest stages of placement whether the catheter is following the right direction, that is, entering the vena cava.

The application of the ECG technique and "Tip navigation" do not require dedicated vascular catheters and can be used with any type of central venous catheter.

SHERLOCK®

The system allows controlled navigation throughout the catheter pathway only dedicated catheters since electromagnetic tracking is used. Like its predecessor, it is capable of simultaneously showing the two ECG traces, basal and intracavitary, assigning a numerical value to the P wave facilitating the operator's task in recognizing the wave with maximal amplitude. However, it does not recognize P wave in patients with atrial fibrillation.

Numerous other systems are on the market that have been more or less successful.

The ultrasound technique combined with tip navigation and tip localization systems provides the best cost-benefit ratio.

As with any technique, to obtain the maximum cost-effectiveness from tip navigation, one needs the following:

- A rational choice of material, methods, human resources, and environment
- Adequate assessment and planning
- The entrusting of the maneuver to trained personnel
- An appropriate logistical organization

Management of Catheter-Related Complications

The main complications related to the placement of central venous catheters, in addition to malpositioning and dislocation, are catheter infections, catheter-related systemic infections, occlusions of the device, and thrombosis of the vessel that houses the catheter.

Infections

Two acronyms, CLABSI and CRBSI, are used to define catheter-related bacteremia:

CLABSI is an epidemiologic definition and is identified as a primary bloodstream infection (bacteremia) in patients to whom a central venous catheter was applied more than 48 hours before the onset of infection and was in situ on or before the day of infection.

CRBSI is the clinical definition of catheter-related bacteremia; it is identified when, in addition to positive blood culture, there are concurrent positive quantitative cultures of the catheter tip for the same pathogen with the same resistance profile, or when in addition to positive blood culture there is a "differential time to positivity—DTTP" (i.e., a difference in the time between collection and positivity of blood cultures taken from the central catheter and those taken from the peripheral routes) equal to or greater than 2 hours. It should also be specified that the 2-hour DTTP criterion is not considered reliable for *Staphylococcus aureus* and *Candida* spp.

Central line-associated bloodstream infection (CLABSI) may increase antibiotic exposure, hospital stay, health care costs, and risk of death. In fact, an updated meta-analysis including18 studies showed an increased risk of death among patients with CLABSI compared with those without this infection. Therefore, it is not surprising that substantial efforts have been made over the past 20 years by various governmental, health care, and professional organizations to sponsor and promote evidence-based guidelines for CLABSI prevention strategies.

Prevention of Catheter-Related Infection

Numerous moments of catheter management can prove to be dangerous sources for infection: very specific rules must be followed to prevent infection.

- Hand hygiene

Surgical washing preferably with alcohol gel and use of sterile gloves.

- Antisepsis of the exit site and/or access point

Chlorhexidine 2% in alcohol solution: antiseptic of first choice if the patient has no intolerance or allergy to chlorhexidine, if the skin around the exit site is intact, and if the catheter is compatible with alcohol solutions. Drying time is 30″.

Iodopovidone 10% in aqueous solution: if the patient is sensitive to chlorhexidine, if the skin around the exit site is not intact, and if the catheter is not compatible with alcohol solutions. Drying time is 2′.

For the application of alcohol-based solutions, the back and forth (forward-backward) technique is indicated, with decidedly short drying time (30 seconds); this technique must be accompanied by vigorous friction of the skin to allow the antiseptic to penetrate the layers of the epidermis reducing the resident microbial flora.

Aqueous-based antiseptics, such as iodopovidone, require, for thorough antisepsis of the skin, the use of a centrifugal circular motion, starting from the center (near the exit site) and moving toward the periphery, without ever going over the same spot again. The operation is to be repeated three times with the use of different gauze/pads each time. There is no emphasis on pressure, but on replacing the pad in each of the consecutive passes. This type of technique is necessary with aqueous-based antiseptics, which take longer to dry (2 minutes), to prevent reintroduction of microorganisms into previously cleaned areas.

The use of 2% chlorhexidine in 70% hydroalcoholic solution (isopropyl alcohol), preferably colored, with a sterile, single-use, single-dose applicator is strongly recommended (no-touch technique).

- Fixation systems

Careful fixation of vascular access prevents dislodgement and reduces infectious, thrombotic, and extravasation risk.

Fixation of venous catheters with sutures should be avoided. There are different types of stitchless fixation systems (sutureless device) specially designed for this function. The frequency of replacement is defined based on the indications in the data sheet; generally, it corresponds to once a week and whenever the system becomes detached or dirty.

- Dressing

The dressing of choice is transparent, breathable sterile adhesive polyurethane film as it allows continuous visual inspection of the insertion site allowing early detection of redness, blood or serum loss, or any extravasation. Chlorhexidine slow-release dressings should be reserved for nontunneled central venous accesses (PICCs, CVCs, FICCs) particularly high-risk patients such as immunocompromised patients, those on high-dose cortisone therapy, and those with previous catheter-related infections or recent implantation of prostheses (valvular or endovascular). Their replacement, like transparent semipermeable dressings, is every 7 days.

- Added devices

Added devices include extensions, filters, valved connectors, simple plugs, and taps. What they have in common, in addition to sterility, is the presence of the luer lock that ensures stability of the system, preventing accidental disconnection and contamination of sterile parts.

Before connecting any device, thorough disinfection of the entry site using sterile gauze soaked in 2% chlorhexidine alcohol with vigorous friction for at least 15″ is mandatory.

- Maintenance

Whenever it is necessary to manipulate a central venous line, it is essential to resort to hand disinfection preferably with alcohol gel, the use of sterile gloves, and chlorhexidine-soaked gauze disinfection of the adjunct fittings and devices.

Suspected Systemic Catheter-Related Infection

Tip culture examination should not be routinely performed at the end of CVC use. In case there are signs of systemic infection in the presence of a central venous catheter since tip culture examination necessarily requires the sacrifice of the device, it is advisable to proceed with device removal only in selected cases and in the presence of signs and symptoms of severe sepsis since international guidelines indicate that it is possible to arrive at a definite diagnosis of CRBSI using the paired culture method (DTTP), without removal of the catheter.

Instead, it is always indicated to perform blood cultures, as per procedures defined in the specific scopes, taking samples from ALL lumens of the central device and peripheral route at the same time, with specific request to the microbiology laboratory so that DTTP can be defined.

In case of confirmed catheter-related sepsis, it will be the clinician's choice whether to proceed with catheter removal or choose antibiotic strategies aimed at device rescue based on the isolated microorganism and antibiogram, proceeding in selected cases with antibiotic lock prescription or removal along with systemic therapy.

The most serious systemic complications are systemic infections, referred to in the literature as catheter-related bloodstream infection (CRBSI) or central line-associated bloodstream infection (CLABSI).

We speak of CRBSI when the source of the infectious outbreak is the CVC itself: in this situation, the pathogen isolated in the blood is the same as that isolated from the CVC.

In contrast, we speak of CVC-associated bacteremia (CLABSI) when this correlation cannot be documented with certainty, that is, when the same pathogen cannot be isolated, but the CVC remains the only plausible focus.

CRBSIs, associated with CVC implantation and management, are among the most potentially dangerous care-related complications.

For a correct diagnosis of CVC-related infection, it is essential to integrate the clinic of infection (evaluating signs and symptoms such as fever, hypotension, skin redness, discharge, etc.) with microbiological and laboratory data.

The diagnostic gold standard in this case is blood cultures performed simultaneously from both peripheral vein and central catheter as per specific company procedures. Correctly performing blood cultures and sending blood draws to microbiology according to the recommended timeframes and request procedures turn out to be of paramount importance to avoid unnecessary device removals and diagnostic errors.

Catheter Occlusions and/or Vessel Thrombosis

CVC occlusions can be complete, preventing both aspiration and infusion, or partial, allowing infusion, sometimes with increased resistance, but not aspiration.

The main causes of partial occlusion are the following:

- Kinking of the catheter
- Fibrin sleeve (a kind of veil that occludes the lumen at the tip only on aspiration)
- Thrombosis of the tip
- Malposition

Occlusions recognize intraluminal causes and extraluminal causes.

Extraluminal causes are usually recognizable at the level of the infusion line connections or at mispositioning of the Huber needle (Port).

Intraluminal causes recognize mechanical, chemical, or thrombotic causes. Mechanical causes are kneeling, dislocation, and adhesion to the inner vessel wall. Chemical causes depend on crystallization of precipitates due to chemically and physically incompatible simultaneous infusions or sequential infusions without adequate flushing with 0.9% NaCl solution (at least 20 mL) by flush technique. Recall, in this regard, that irritating, stinging, vesicant substances with osmolarity >900 mOsm and pH <5 and >9 must necessarily be infused centrally. Thrombotic causes may extend more or less to the catheter lumen or affect the vessel. In such a case, the risk is that of central vessel thrombosis with the possibility of pulmonary embolism, which can also prove fatal to the patient.

Intraluminal occlusion may be due to inadequate/ineffective lavage, inadequate intraluminal flow, frequent withdrawals, or blood reflux.

This complication is frequently due to a mix of coagulated blood and drug precipitates and is often iatrogenic (inadequate flushing and lock).

Fibroblast sheath occlusion, a sleeve of collagen and fibroblasts, occurs as a reaction due to the presence of a foreign body in the blood. Often asymptomatic, it can result in partial or total occlusion. When occlusion is partial, the catheter infuses but does not aspirate, and overflow at the exit site may result.

Thrombotic occlusion occurs as a result of damage to the endothelium: the process extends and also involves the tip of the venous catheter, covering its surface and limiting its functionality. This situation can be determined because of the trauma generated during insertion, the reason for which placement by micropuncture technique is recommended, in the presence of reduced blood flow due to the presence of an incongruous ratio between catheter lumen and vessel lumen, due to malpositioning of the tip or due to hypercoagulability related to certain pathologies.

Prevention of Thrombosis

Prevention of occlusion is based on an adequate flushing (flush) protocol with physiologic saline, by syringe operated with push/pause technique, before and after each infusion followed by closure of the system (lock). Flushes with 10 mL of saline are recommended, preferably with prefilled syringes at neutral pressure under normal conditions, increasing the volume to 20 mL after withdrawals, infusion of blood or blood products, parenteral nutrition with lipids, and MDC injection. The use of heparinized solutions has no evidence of efficacy and should be avoided.

Other preventive interventions include the use of neutral pressure NFC valved connectors in order to prevent reflux of blood into the catheter. In situations where it is not possible to take advantage of the action of NFCs (e.g., when removing the Huber needle from a Port), maneuvers that leave positive pressure within the system should be used; in addition, simultaneous infusion of incompatible drugs should be avoided. Information regarding incompatibilities should be carefully sought by operators.

Catheter Unblocking Maneuver

In general, after ruling out vessel thrombosis or other causes (e.g., mechanical malfusion), catheter rescue is preferable to catheter removal. To perform this maneuver correctly, one needs to be very familiar with the physical characteristics of the device.

The maneuver is called the three-way tap system (Fig. 5.8).

We need a three-way tap, two 10-mL luer-lock syringes, 0.9% NaCl solution, and deconstricting solution, usually urokinase at increasing concentrations (5000 I.U./mL; 10,000 I.U./mL).

The method consists of connecting the three-way tap prefilled with saline to the catheter and turning the tap valve to open the pathway between the empty syringe and the CVC. Keeping the syringe suctioned, turn the faucet valve so that the pathways between the syringe with the deostruent solution and the catheter are open and connected; in this way, the catheter will suck in some of the solution because of the negative pressure created by the previous maneuver. The operation is repeated every 3–5 minutes so that a few milliliters of the deostruent solution can be inserted into the catheter and the aspiration with empty syringe corresponds to the reflux of blood into the catheter. Allow the deostruent solution to work for at least 4–6 hours, and if necessary, repeat with more concentrated solution. In this case, investigate the outcome of the maneuver only after 12 hours.

If unsuccessful, consider removal of the catheter.

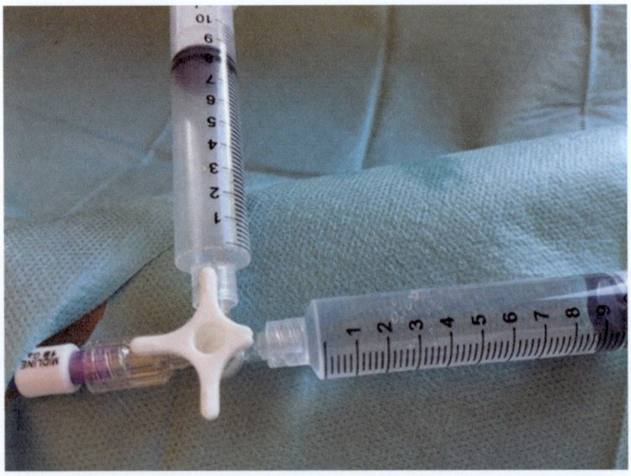

Fig. 5.8 Three-way tap system

Deep Venous Thrombosis

Catheter-related thrombosis (CRT) refers to the presence, in the catheter-traveled section of vein, of venous thrombosis caused by endothelial damage. Blood stasis and hypercoagulability (Virchow's triad) also contribute to its occurrence. The incidence of CRT ranges from 1% to 66%, depending on the type of population, different diagnostic modalities (echocolordoppler, AngioTC), and different types of devices included in epidemiologic studies. The population most prone to develop CRT is cancer patients, and the device most prone to determine CRT is the central catheter placed in the femoral vein. The evolution of CRT can include pulmonary embolism, sometimes fatal. CRT is frequently asymptomatic; when symptomatic, the signs and symptoms are due to venous flow obstruction, and some of the signs may include pain, edema, erythema in the extremities, neck, shoulder, or chest, and superficial venous circles.

After careful study with AngioTC to assess the extent of thrombosis quantify undertake anticoagulation therapy as soon as possible in consultation with the attending, if not contraindicated. If the catheter is found to be functional and well placed, it can be used regularly; otherwise, anticoagulation therapy with EBPM at a coagulant dosage should still be started before removal. In cases where there is suspicion of septic thrombosis, the risk of clinical deterioration related to infection makes timely removal of the device reasonable in contrast, despite the fact that there is an increased risk of pulmonary embolism due to mobilization of pericatheter thrombotic material.

Catheter Rupture

Rupture can occur in the inner (not visible) or outer tract (with immediate diagnosis).

Suspicion of catheter rupture is raised if there are signs and symptoms such as leakage at the insertion site, catheter malfunction (e.g., inability to aspirate blood, frequent infusion pump alarms, and resistance to flushing), infraclavicular pain and/or swelling along the catheter pathway during infusion, and paresthesias. If a catheter rupture with risk of catheter embolization is suspected, prompt action needs to be taken. Diagnostic confirmation of catheter damage and catheter rupture or embolization is placed by radiological techniques (X-ray or CT scan of the chest and fluoroscopic examination) or ultrasound. If part of the embolized catheter is present, its removal by interventional radiology/cardiology procedures is planned.

Most of the preps currently on the market withstand infusion pressures up to 300 Psi. They are referred to as power injectable. Ruptures are more pronounced with silicone catheters than with the latest generation of polyurethane catheters. Any power injectable CVC can be used for infusion of iodinated contrast medium as long as the pressure limit of the automatic injectors is set at 300 Psi.

Bibliography

1. Le buone pratiche per gli accessi vascolari SIAARTI. 2018.
2. Chaves F, Garnacho-Montero J, Del Pozo JL, Bouza E, Capdevila JA, de Cueto M, Domínguez MÁ, Esteban J, FernÁndez-Hidalgo N, FernÁndez Sampedro M, Fortún J, Guembe M, Lorente L, Paño JR, Ramírez P, Salavert M, SÁnchez M, Vallés J. Diagnosis and treatment of catheter-related bloodstream infection: clinical guidelines of the Spanish Society of Infectious Diseases and Clinical Microbiology and (SEIMC) and the Spanish Society of Spanish Society of Intensive and Critical Care Medicine and Coronary Units (SEMICYUC). Med Intensiva (Engl Ed). 2018;42(1):5–36.
3. O'Grady NP. Prevention of central line–associated bloodstream infections. N Engl J Med. 2023;389:1121–31. https://doi.org/10.1056/NEJMra2213296.
4. Protocollo di gestione degli accessi vascolari nei pazienti adulti. Commissione Regionale Dispositivi Medici, Regione Emilia-Romagna; 2019.
5. Chen P, Zhu B, Wan G, Qin L. The incidence of asymptomatic thrombosis related to peripherally inserted central catheter in adults: a systematic review and meta-analysis people's. Nurs Open. 2021;8(5):2249–61. https://doi.org/10.1002/nop2.811. Epub 2021 Feb 22. PMID: 33617142; PMCID: PMC8363368.

6 Long-Term Central Venous Access

Della Vigna

Indications for Long-Term Central Venous Access

A precise definition of "long-term" is difficult. An arbitrary time for any central venous catheter with a planned duration of use greater than 6 weeks is probably a reasonable definition [1, 2]. Indications for such tools have been listed since late 1990s [3]; however with more recent advances in treatment of a growing numbers of medical conditions, long-term central venous access should be considered in any case of need for prolonged infusions especially when venous access are poor. The different conditions that may more frequently require a long-term venous catheter are summarized in Table 6.1.

A further parameter deserving attention to give a correct indication for long-term central venous catheter placement is the scenario in which the device will be used. Inpatients are more likely candidates to have an intensive venous devices maintenance from nurse staff as well as for homecare assisted patients. Outpatients with a sporadic need for a venous access will benefit more of a reliable infusion system with a complete subcutaneous placement. Lastly, costs have to be mentioned: "which catheter will result in the best outcome at the least cost?" is the correct question asked since more than two decades [4]. The answer suggested has taken the lead becoming the gold standard until now: "Significant cost savings and

Table 6.1 Indications for long-term venous catheter

Cancer chemotherapy	Oncologic patients
Hemato-oncological disorders	Pediatric-adult patients with liquid malignancies
Long-term antibiotic treatments	Bacterial endocarditis, cystic fibrosis
Hemodialysis	Fistula exhaustion
Repeated blood transfusions	Hematological patients
Total parental nutrition	Small bowel syndrome, malabsorption

D. Vigna (✉)
Unit for Research and Development of Technologies in Interventional Oncology, Division of Interventional Radiology, European Institute of Oncology, Milan, Italy
e-mail: paolo.dellavigna@ieo.it

R. Lanocita, M. Lamperti (eds.), *Practical Guide to Central Venous Cannulation*,
https://doi.org/10.1007/978-3-031-90326-7_6

fewer severe complications can be realized by preferential use of peripherally inserted central catheters when clinically indicated (PICC)." Such a tool has been shown to have so much advantages (see below) that often its placement has been reported as over-indicated [5, 6]. However, as usual, a correct tool care is the key for a longer duration in order to avoid several placements instead.

Types of Long-Term Central Venous Access Devices, Including Ports and Tunneled Catheters

A further principle that could be used to specify how long does "long-term" mean is more easily to define the kind of device selected for the access. Planning an infusional or supportive care longer than 4–5 weeks should imply the use of one long-term device since the beginning depending on the supposed duration:

1. Time-limit devices: all the catheters implanted with the proximal extremity emerging from the skin have a time of expiration. Several technical strategies have been invented to maintain a longer dwell time:
   - Tunneling: the catheter shaft does not appear directly from the skin puncturing site but is "tunneled" more distant trough the subcutaneous layer emerging further away. Such trick ensures a more protective action against bacterial colonization reaching the vessel lumen. This technique requires a special attention for catheter removal being aware the vein puncture point on which apply pressure for hemostasis is different from the poking out point of the catheter.
   - Cuffed catheters: tissue growth into the cuff anchors it after about 3 weeks and is a barrier to the tracking of skin microorganisms along the catheter. Often tunneled catheters also have a Dacron cuff: an antimicrobial cuff surrounding the catheter near the entry site, which is coated in antimicrobial solution.
   - Valved (Groshong) catheters: it has a slit-like orifice adjacent to the distal end which functions as a valve. It stops blood back flow, prevents air entry with negative intrathoracic pressure (see Chap. 7 for air embolism), and does not require heparin lock infusion. A difference in pressure is required either by suction or injection to open the valve. A Groshong catheter is recognizable at a glance by its labeling blue color and absence of an external clamp. The real negative feature is the cost.
   - PICCs (peripherally inserted central catheters): these catheters are usually inserted at the bedside via an antecubital vein and are available with single or multiple lumina. Basically, the peripheral approach reduces the risk of central access complications (hematomas, pneumothorax). With a proper training, it can be performed under ultrasound guidance by nurses. The tip is nevertheless advanced until right atrium or superior-inferior vena cava depending on its specific purpose, offering all the advantages of a central line. Drawbacks are a higher thrombosis and occlusion rate due to their narrow lumens and reduced flow rates [7] and the susceptibility to tip relocation in case of arm movement. The real benefit of such a device is the full management by nurses and the possibility for trained operators to correctly deploy the line without X-ray assistance. This allow both biological and economic advantages. In-site duration has been a matter of debate: if this device is useful for any treatment longer than 5 days, thrombotic complications of superficial venous system can easily evolve to the central venous system causing consequences similar to classical central venous lines [8]. Moreover, bloodstream infections have more recently been found to be higher than expected [9], suggesting a limitation in the PICC's dwell time to 25 days, even for inhospital patients. These criticisms have led to guidelines that largely limit PICC

use and reduce its recommended dwell time [10, 11]. Since then, PICCs have more appropriately been referred to as mid-term central access devices.

Different configurations of the described issues can be adopted to increase safety and permanence times: Valved catheters for jugular and subclavian access have been designed with specific Dacron cuff and the possibility of tunneling. With such a combination, a central venous access in good maintenance conditions can last even 6 months. However, the same option for PICCs has not been endorsed by guidelines even if occasionally reported [12]. In particular, valved devices could allow to a significant rise in PICC's cost reducing significantly such device affordability. Finally, a simple consideration about catheter materials could be noteworthy: While short-term access is commonly made from polyurethane, making them stiff enough to insert over a guidewire, long-term is largely made with more flexible materials such as silicone to reduce vessel damage and thrombosis.

2. Totally implantable devices (port): those devices are hypothetically designed to last longer in reason of their complete subcutaneous placement. The complete isolation from bacteria colonization is the key to guarantee an infusional line time as long as possible. Usually, the catheter is connected to a reservoir with a small silicone septum that is possible to puncture from the outside with a dedicated needle (Huber needle). This is a specific noncoring needle with a hole on the side of the tip not to permanently damage the silicone septum. Once the needle is in place, the infusional line can be used for the planned therapy. However, the longer the needle stays in place, the higher the possibility of bacterial colonization and subsequent infections. Port placement is a little more invasive than tunneled catheters or PICCs; after the central venous cannulation, a limited 2–3 cm skin incision is needed for the reservoir pocket with a consequent healing time and a final scar. Reservoir dimensions should be a compromise: not too big for patient's comfort and cosmetics concerns, but not too small allowing its easy detection for needle puncturing. Some port manufacturers provide devices of different size not only for pediatric purpose. In patients with high BMI, indeed a normal dimension reservoir could not be easy to detect for the needle sticking
   - Pros: the main advantage for the patient is the lack of limitations. After a few days, once a reliable scar has formed, it is possible to resume normal activities without concerns about dislocation or damage. This feature makes ports the ideal devices for patients requiring several infusions in a long outpatient time lapse. Cancer treatments are the most frequent indication for this kind of central venous access.
   - Cons: the longer procedural time and the scar left are the main patient concerns. Device cost is clearly higher than external devices. However, the main pitfall is the need for device removal in case of complication. Septic or nonseptic complications (see below) may require port explant even without the possibility of using the same vessel for a further access.

For totally implantable long-term venous access materials, to guarantee a proper functionality as well as patient comfort is a continuous challenge. Most of the manufacturers' effort relies on materials with anti-thrombogenic and anti-infectious properties to avoid the most frequent complications after a long indwelling. The ideal catheter should be soft enough not to cause endothelial damage but stable and chemically inert not causing thrombosis or infection. Up to now, no rubber material fulfils all these requirements. Nowadays, catheter materials frequently consist of polyurethane or silicon rubber materials. However, a constant research of new solution to reduce infection and thrombosis is running [13, 14]. The other reason why port cost is higher than that of tunneled or nontunneled catheters is because placement is performed by medical personnel, while for catheters, specific nurse training could be sufficient. Most important than device placement is however its maintenance and its care. For both totally and nontotally implantable devices, the most feared complication is infection. Nursing attentions are of paramount importance in order to ensure the device is in place as long as possible without consequences. For such a purpose, even practical details that can be considered meticulous are strongly suggested:

- Environment should be checked for a proper clean scenario when the line is in use.
- Hand washing.
- Proximal hub should always be covered with specific locks in external devices when not in use.
- A daily check should evaluate the proper functionality of the line and signs of infection, including erythema.
- Bandage changing should be as frequent as required depending on the site/scar conditions. In normal conditions, a sterile transparent dressing could last from 2 to 5 days, but in case of partial detachment or integrity failure, changing should be immediate.
- A sterile environment is requested for Huber needle placement. That means sterile gloves, sterile field on the cutaneous access site (either 70% alcohol or chlorhexidine), and sterile drape.
- If external catheter management is allowed with nonsterile gloves, connections of infusion lines require sterile precautions.

Insertion Techniques and Management of Complications Associated with Long-Term Devices

Introduction

As already specified, central venous port has been used for administering intravenous medications and nutritional support that cannot be given safely through peripheral venous catheters. The number of placements has been increasing mainly due to the increase in the number of patients with cancer who require long-term treatments [15].

Careful preoperative assessment is advised. Before performing port placement, patient (age, gender, underlying illness, medical history, height, and weight) and test data (blood data and imaging findings) information should be collected. Reported patient-specific risk factors for the onset of central vein puncture complications include obesity (body mass index (BMI) >30), underweight (emaciation, BMI <20), edema, blood coagulation disorder, pacemaker, surgical wound at the puncture site, respiratory function disorder, and a history of previous failures in the insertion of CVCs [16].

An informed consent must be obtained from the patient, explaining the advantages and the risks of the individual patient associated with catheterization.

Contraindications such as a severe coagulation disorders (thrombocytes <50/nL, partial thromboplastin time (PTT) <50%, international normalized ration (INR) >1.5), systemic or local infection, or known allergy to the materials or contrast agent must be excluded beforehand. Since there is no agreement on the usefulness of using antibiotic prophylaxis to prevent catheter colonization, before insertion, it is not usually recommended [17, 18].

The procedure is to be performed at a location where aseptic manipulation can be ensured such as in an operating theater or angiography room. Monitoring of the patient is necessary; thus, any mechanical complications that occur due to puncturing (bleeding, pneumothorax, hemopneumothorax, arrhythmia, airway obstruction due to hematoma, cerebral infarction, etc.) can be discovered quickly and treated as soon as possible. It requires monitoring of peripheral arterial oxygen saturation (pulse oximeter), electrocardiography, and arterial blood pressure.

Maximal sterile barrier precautions are fundamental. The operator must wear a mask, cap (covering all the hair), sterile gloves, and a sterile gown, and the patient is covered with large sterile drapes. Disinfection of the skin is performed with a 0.5% chlorhexidine preparation with alcohol. If there is a contraindication to chlorhexidine, tincture of iodine, an iodophor, or 70% alcohol can be used as alternatives.

The percutaneous approach to the subclavian or internal jugular vein currently is the most popular procedure for placing central venous catheters. The Centers for Disease Control recommends not to use routinely venous cut-down procedures as a method to insert catheters, even for long-term ones, because percutaneously placed catheters are associated with a lower infection rate than surgically implanted ones [19]. However, in neonates and in children, not routinely but in selected cases, venous cut-down might be the safest choice.

The insertion of a central venous catheter requires access to a tributary vein of the vena cava. The most commonly used approach involves positioning the catheter in a large vein of the neck (internal jugular vein), upper thorax (subclavian vein), or groin (femoral vein). There is insufficient evidence to recommend a specific insertion site, but the femoral vein should be avoided unless there is a contraindication to the other sites (e.g., SVC syndrome), due to the increased risk of infection and concerns about thrombosis [20].

Insertion Techniques

Traditionally, anatomical landmarks on the body's surface and ultrasound are used to locate the correct plane for catheter insertion. Anatomic variations and the presence of venous thrombosis can hardly be identified using a landmark technique. In contrast, ultrasound offers numerous and indisputable advantages: the ability to visualize underlying structures in the thorax, neck, and extremities leads to greater success, speed, and safety in all vascular access procedures. For these reasons, the use of ultrasound has become the standard of care in central venous access [16, 21]. Using ultrasound guidance to place central venous catheters has been demonstrated to decrease the number of insertion attempts, time to cannulation, and complications of central venous catheterization [22].

The choice of vessel should not be based only on the operator's preference, but should be the result of an examination of the patient's clinical condition. The percutaneous approach to the subclavian vein or internal jugular vein is currently the most popular procedure. Evaluating potential risk factors for difficult catheterization is essential, such as skeletal deformity, presence of scars, obesity, or history of previous surgery at the insertion site. The use of ultrasound can assist the operator in selecting the vessel by assessing its patency or abnormalities such as thrombosis, stenosis, external compression, anatomical variations in size and shape, and in choosing the needle path, by examining adjacent structures that should be avoided, such as arteries, nerves, and pleura.

US probes best suited for CVC placement are small linear array probes with high-frequency transducers (5–15 MHz). These probes usually have a scanning surface of about 20–50 mm providing a good resolution for visualizing superficial structures and the vasculature, making it ideal for identifying the internal jugular vein or subclavian vein during central venous catheter placement. In some cases, a curvilinear probe with low-frequency transducers (3–5 MHz) may also be used, particularly for deeper veins or in obese patients. 2D imaging (complemented by Doppler US functions) is currently the standard technique used for US-guided central venous access. All US probes have an index mark (a small physical notch on one side of the probe) that corresponds with an orientation marker on one side of the US scan sector shown on the US device screen and thus helps to obtain the correct probe orientation during US examination. US machines should have the ability to record and save US images and loops for clinical documentation (and teaching purposes) [23].

There is no preferred side, unless there are clinical contraindications such as upper limb edema secondary to axillary lymph node dissection, presence of adenopathies, or rotational flaps within reconstructive head and neck surgery. A three-arm randomized trial showed that the central venous access insertion site does not influence early or late occurrence of complications of these devices, at least when implanted in an experienced environment [24].

Proper orientation of the ultrasound probe is crucial for adequate visualization of both the vein and the needle. The operator can choose to visualize the target vessel using a longitudinal (long-axis view) or transverse (short-axis view) axis.

With the transverse axis, the probe is oriented perpendicular to the vein and displays a cross-sectional view of the vessel, and both the target vessel and adjacent vessels can be seen, but only a portion of the needle will be visible as it passes under the transducer, and the needle tip cannot be continuously visualized.

With the longitudinal axis, the probe is aligned parallel to the vein. The operator can view the target vessel, allowing for better assessment of the entire length of the vein. While observing both the target vein and the needle, the needle can be visualized in real time as it approaches the vein, making it easier to direct it into the vessel along its entire trajectory. The ability to visualize the needle from the insertion point to the vessel allows for puncturing only the anterior wall, reducing the number of puncture attempts.

Although there is insufficient evidence to recommend a specific insertion site for cannulation, access through the subclavian vein appears to have a lower incidence of complications and a higher patient preference [25].

The most commonly used technique involves a modified Seldinger approach with the insertion of a guidewire into the superior vena cava and further through the right atrium into the inferior vena cava to assure venous puncture; the puncture tract is dilated with a detachable sheath dilator. The catheter is introduced into the superior vena cava through the peel away sheath [26]. In port placement, the catheter tip should ideally be positioned in the superior vena cava (SVC) or just at the junction where the SVC meets the right atrium. This placement helps ensure optimal flow and reduces the risk of complications such as thrombosis or catheter-related infections. Several methods are used to measure depth of catheter insertion including electrocardiogram guidance method. However, proper imaging guidance, such as fluoroscopy, is the more precise method used to confirm the correct placement during the procedure [27].

Once the catheter is positioned correctly, a pocket is prepared for the reservoir. The incision on the skin is made approximately three to four centimeters below the catheter access site. The pocket is prepared by exposing the fascia of the pectoral muscle. At this point, with a tunneling device, a subcutaneous tunnel for the catheter is established and the catheter is connected to the reservoir, which is then placed in the pocket and secured to the pectoralis major muscle fascia with sutures. The pocket is closed with absorbable subcutaneous sutures and tissue adhesive at the skin level (Fig. 6.1).

Finally, the reservoir is punctured with a Huber needle to test the proper functioning of the system, and fluoroscopy is used to check the system's integrity, the catheter's course, and its tip position (Fig. 6.2).

Complications and Their Management

Central venous access devices (CVADs) are critical for effective and efficient management of patients because they facilitate urgent, acute, or prolonged access to the bloodstream for the administration of prescribed and supportive therapies and repeated blood sampling [28, 29]. However, they also present considerable risk of complications and many are removed prematurely before the end of prescribed therapy.

Central venous access complications significantly increase length of stay and healthcare costs and negatively impact the quality of life. Many complications are preventable with improved training and meticulous technique, and growing awareness of these issues has led to even greater emphasis on addressing these deficiencies.

The complications of CVCs can be classified into two main categories: early (intraoperative and postimplantion period to first use) and late complications.

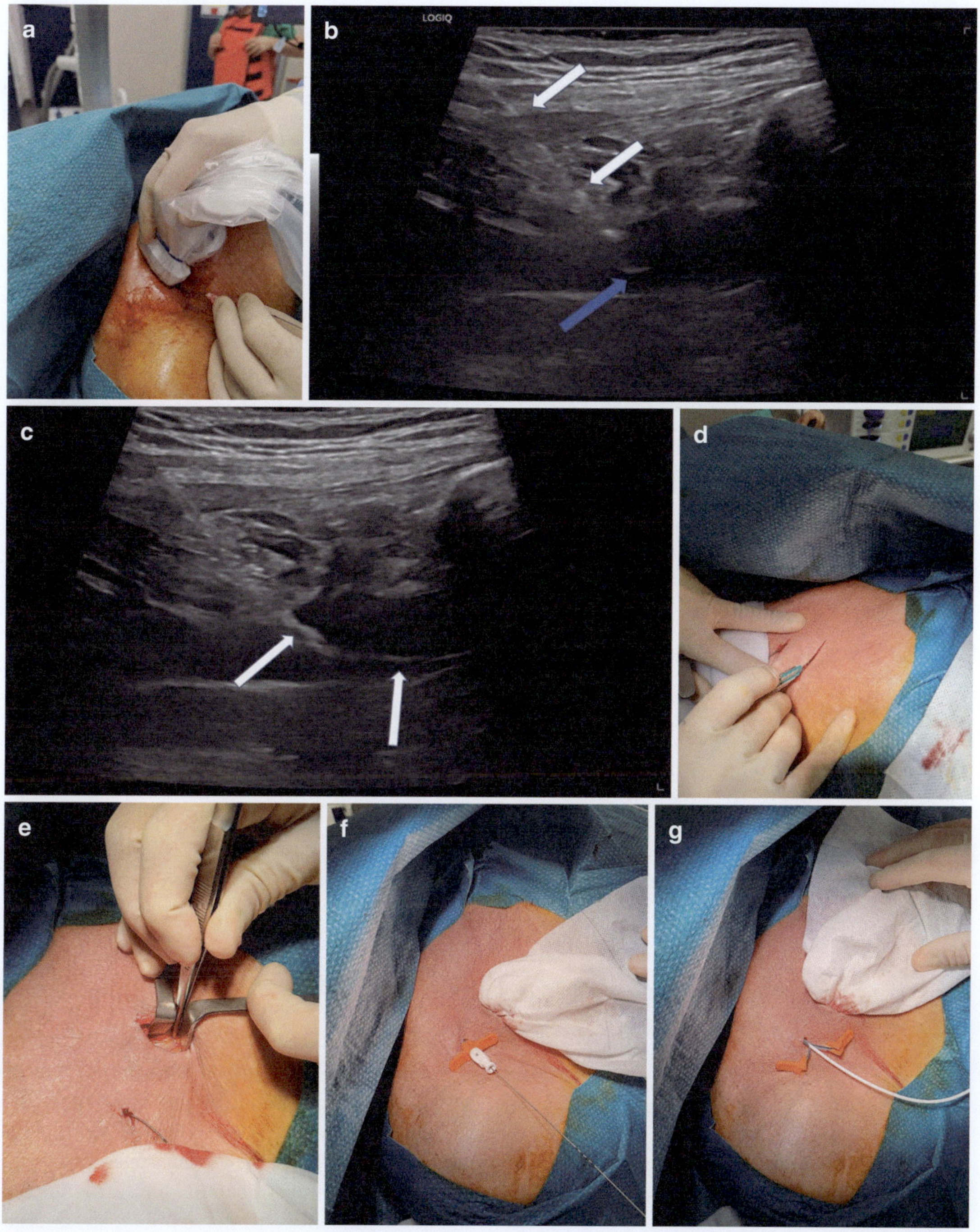

Fig. 6.1 The probe is positioned longitudinally along the subclavian sulcus (**a**), and the needle is inserted along its long axis. Ultrasound (**b**) facilitates needle visualization (white arrows) along its pathway, with the tip (blue arrow) located within the vein and the guidewire (**c**) inserted into the vein. After inserting the metal guide, an incision is made approximately three to four centimeters caudal to the access point (**d**). A pocket is then created to accommodate the reservoir (**e**). The puncture tract is dilated using a detachable sheath dilator (**f**). The catheter is introduced into the superior vena cava through the peel-away sheath (**g**). The catheter is tunneled (**h**) and connected to the reservoir (**i**), which is anchored to the fascia of the pectoral muscle (**l**). The pocket is closed with absorbable subcutaneous sutures (**m**) and tissue adhesive at the skin level (**n**)

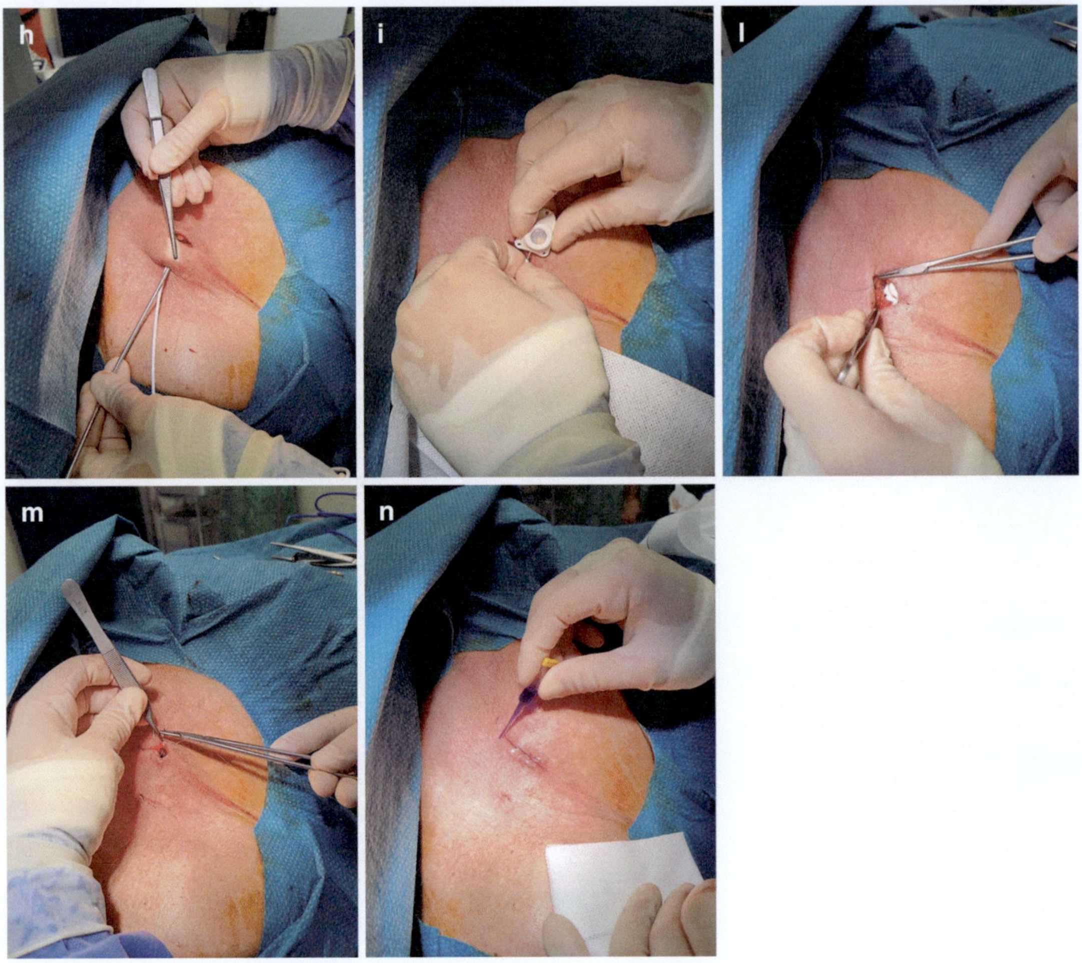

Fig. 6.1 (continued)

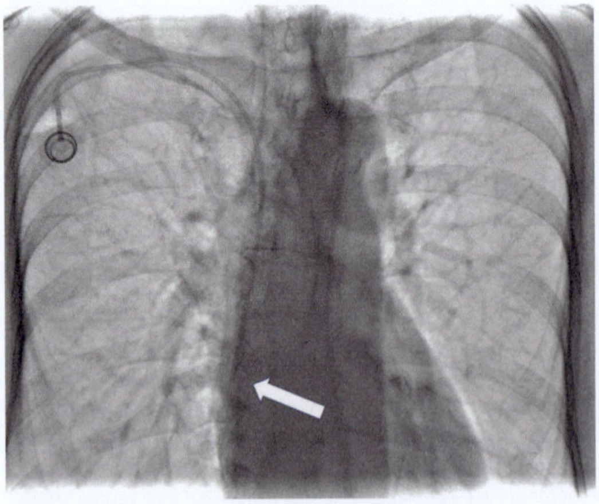

Fig. 6.2 Fluoroscopy performed at the end of the procedure confirmed the integrity of the system, the catheter's path, and the position of its tip near the atriocaval junction (white arrow)

Early Complications

Early complications are defined as complications occurring during the implantation procedure or within the first 24 h after implantation and complications developed 24 h to 30 days after implantation procedure. They include pneumothorax, hemothorax, primary malposition, arrhythmias, air embolism, iatrogenic nerve injury, and arterial perforation causing clinically relevant bleeding. Some minor mechanical complications (minor bleeding, self-limiting arrhythmia, and nonpersistent nerve injury) normally do not affect the patient, but others (arterial puncture, failed catheterization, and catheter tip malposition) may force postponement of surgery and chemotherapy. Major mechanical complications (major bleeding, arterial catheterization, symptomatic arrhythmia, pneumothorax, and persistent nerve injury) typically require acute treatment or invasive intervention, in combination with prolonged observation of the patient.

Pneumothorax is described as the most frequent early complication of percutaneous central vein cannulation, with a prevalence of 0.5–12% depending on differences in clinical features, access site, and operator experience [30].

With the ultrasound-guided approach, pneumothorax has become extremely rare. It has been suggested that postprocedural chest radiographs are not routinely required after image-guided (by fluoroscopy or ultrasound) central venous catheter insertion [31, 32]. A postprocedural chest radiograph can be performed on a case-by-case basis in symptomatic patients or when there is suspected inappropriate catheter tip position.

Treatment of iatrogenic pneumothorax aims at evacuating air from the pleural space and reexpanding the lung. Available therapeutic options include simple observation; aspiration with a catheter, with or without immediate removal of the catheter after pleural air is evacuated; and insertion of a chest tube or tube thoracostomy [33].

The selection of the approach depends on the size of the pneumothorax, the severity of symptoms, and whether there is a persistent air leak or not.

Arrhythmia occurs if the catheter is fed too far and can be corrected by pulling the catheter back.

In case of accidental arterial puncture, a firm pressure for 10 minutes has to be applied, monitoring neurological, hemodynamic, and airways parameters.

In case of hemothorax, a large caliber chest drain must be inserted to drain the blood. However, in cases of massive hemothorax, a surgical approach should be considered.

Air embolism can be managed placing the patient in lateral decubitus and Trendelenburg position, but for a deeper description, refer to Chap. 7 [34–36].

Late Complications

Late complications are defined as complications that develop after 30 days [22]. They are mechanical complications (obstruction, pinch off, fractures, dislodgement, or migration); extravasation injuries; infections (including phlebitis of the cannulated vessel); and catheter and vein thrombosis/occlusion (including deep vein thrombosis, pulmonary embolism, or SVC syndrome).

Mechanical Complications

Obstruction of Central Venous Catheters (CVCs)

Obstruction of a central venous catheter (CVC) is typically due to the intraluminal precipitation of lipid aggregates, drugs, clots, contrast medium, or the formation of a fibrin sleeve. Chest X-ray should be performed to rule out an internal kink or dislocation of the catheter.

Fibrin Sleeve

A fibrin sleeve is a structure formed by the aggregation of fibrin, a protein involved in the clotting process. In the context of medical devices such as central venous catheters, fibrin sleeves can develop around these devices as the body responds to their presence. Postmortem examinations have found fibrin sleeves in 100% of central venous catheters, and they are associated with catheter dysfunction, thrombus formation, and microbial colonization. When access is achieved via the subclavian vein, fibrin sleeve formation can extend from the entry point into the subclavian vein for a variable length, potentially extending beyond the catheter tip and eventually enclosing the catheter completely. Furthermore, the formation of the fibrin sleeve may be exacerbated by continuous movement and mechanical irritation of the vein wall. As the fibrin sleeve extends distally, it can cause catheter dysfunction by creating a flap valve effect, allowing injection while preventing the withdrawal of blood flow, until the catheter is completely occluded and rendered unusable [37].

The best method for detecting a fibrin sheath is through direct contrast material injection into the catheter lumen (i.e., catheter venography). In the absence of a significant fibrin sheath, a straight, uninhibited jet of contrast medium should be observed at the lumen exit site. However, in the presence of a fibrin sheath, the normal ejection of contrast material is disrupted, resulting in a turbulent outflow appearance that can vary. A thin layer of contrast material often refluxes upward between the catheter and the fibrin sheath before escaping into the vein above. If the fibrin sleeve encases the entire intravascular length of the catheter, it may result in contrast material tracking back through the venotomy entry site and extravasating into the surrounding soft tissues or onto the skin (Fig. 6.3) [38].

Flow restoration can be achieved either mechanically or pharmacologically. Mechanical techniques include transfemoral stripping of the

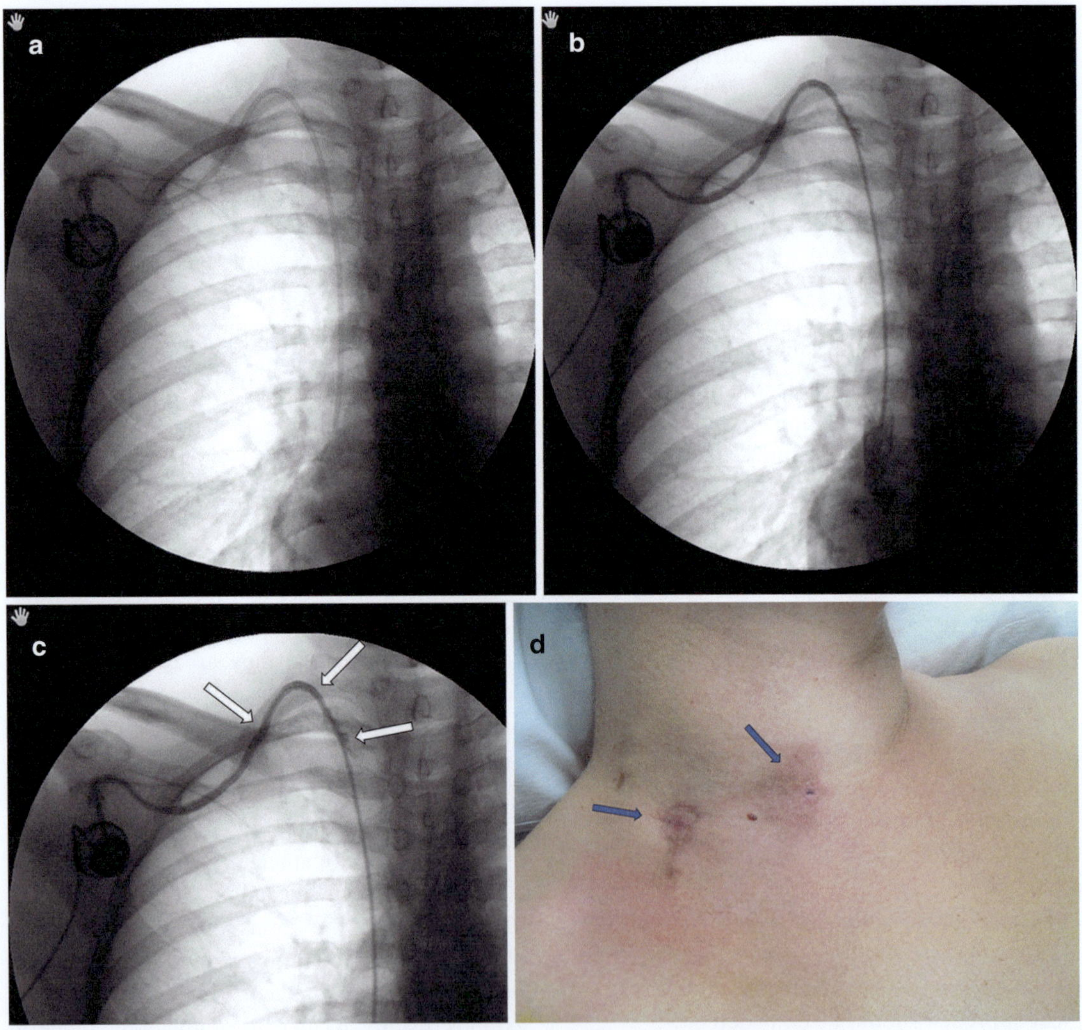

Fig. 6.3 Catheter dysfunction of a right-sided transjugular port (**a**) allowing injection while preventing withdrawal. Control with contrast medium injected through the Huber needle (**b**) reveals a fibrin sleeve encasing the entire length of the catheter, with contrast traveling up the catheter to the subcutaneous tissue (**c**, white arrows). Extravasation of chemotherapy infused through the catheter resulted in damage to the patient's subcutaneous tissue and skin (**d**, blue arrows)

fibrin sheath with a snare or its endoluminal disruption using various devices such as guide wires, catheters, or balloon catheters, the latter technique often involving catheter exchange. Pharmacologic therapy typically involves the use of thrombolytic agents [39].

Pinch-Off Syndrome

Pinch-off syndrome (POS) occurs when a long-term central venous catheter is compressed between the clavicle and the first rib. This compression may lead to malfunction or obstruction and can result in a tear or even complete transection and embolization of the catheter. The clinical presentation of POS is highly variable; patients may exhibit pain, with or without swelling, at the catheter insertion site, or experience catheter dysfunction with difficulty in aspiration or flushing. POS may be preceded by the identification of a "pinch-off sign" on chest X-ray, in which the catheter appears indented as it passes beneath the clavicle (Fig. 6.4). The costoclavicular ligament, a strong band of dense fibrous tissue, connects the first rib to the inferior surface of the medial clavicle. This problem arises when the catheter is inserted medially, crossing the ligament outside the subclavian vein before it penetrates the vessel medially. A properly placed catheter traverses the costoclavicular space within the subclavian vein, which lies in a more capacious region, thereby protecting the catheter from compression. The pinch and friction on the catheter caused by movements of the clavicle and first rib can eventually wear through and transect the catheter tubing. This is a potentially severe complication that can be prevented by avoiding placement via infraclavicular blind venipuncture in favor of ultrasound-guided techniques. If the syndrome is suspected, the catheter must be promptly removed, as should be done for patients with radiographic evidence of catheter compression [40–42].

Catheter Fracture

Fracture of a central venous catheter with subsequent embolization is a rare but potentially serious complication. The distal tip of the embolized catheter can migrate to the pulmonary artery, right ventricle, right atrium, inferior vena cava, superior vena cava, hepatic veins, or a thymic vein. Recognized mechanisms for catheter embolization include disconnection from the port chamber, operator-induced damage during catheter explantation or exchange, catheter clearance techniques, and pinch-off syndrome. Patients experiencing embolization of a percutaneous venous catheter are most commonly asymptomatic. However, they may present with symptoms of catheter malfunction, such as blockage or localized pain and swelling at the site of infusion. Other symptoms

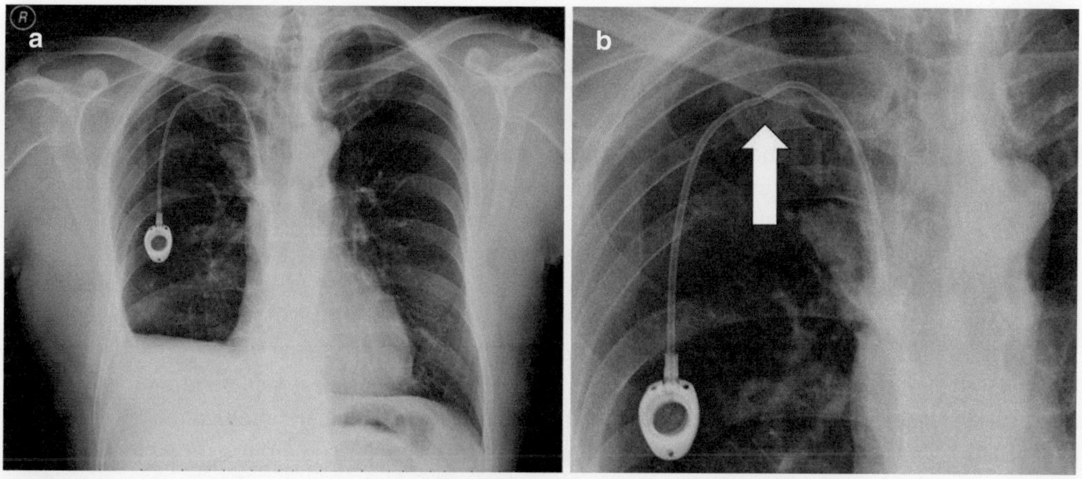

Fig. 6.4 In a right-sided trans-subclavian port (**a**), the catheter may exhibit a narrowing (**b**, white arrow), known as the "pinch-off sign," as it passes between the first rib and the clavicle

can include palpitations, dyspnea, cough, thoracic pain, and septic complications. In most cases, embolized catheters should be removed, and percutaneous endovascular retrieval using a loop snare is the preferred technique [43, 44].

Catheter Dislodgement

Dislodgement and tip migration, also defined as secondary malposition, typically occur when a catheter dislocates due to increased thoracic pressures. The catheter tip may migrate within the jugular vein, subclavian vein, azygos vein, ipsilateral or contralateral mammary vein, thyroid vein, or vertebral vein. If a catheter tip has migrated, the central venous device should not be used due to the risk of infusion into the wrong veins, which can lead to significant complications [45, 46]. This type of complication is primarily attributed to the catheter being too short, with the tip positioned in the upper third of the superior vena cava. In cases of tip migration, repositioning solely by injecting the catheter under pressure is rarely effective. An endovascular approach using a pigtail catheter is generally required, wrapping it around the catheter and attempting to restore its position with gentle traction. This maneuver can also be attempted even if the distal tip is not free, thereby avoiding more complex procedures such as the long loop technique. Unfortunately, the catheter tends to dislocate again, and it is often necessary to remove or replace it [47–49].

Extravasation Injuries

Extravasation is a complication that occurs when intravenous fluid or medication leaks out of the blood vessel into the surrounding tissue. In the context of a central venous catheter, extravasation typically occurs due to catheter malfunction, such as rupture or tear of the catheter or port septum, improper placement, dislodgement, damage to the vein, separation of the catheter from the reservoir, or incorrect placement of the needle into the port septum [50].

Catheter occlusion can be associated with extravasation, as excessive force when flushing the catheter can rupture its connection to the septum [51]. In cancer patients, extravasation of chemotherapeutic vesicant agents can result in significant pain, tissue damage, necrosis, and ulceration. Depending on the site of extravasation, alterations in limb function and even mediastinal damage may occur [52].

Prompt recognition and management are essential to minimize tissue damage and other potential complications. The main symptoms include swelling, redness, and pain at the infusion site; changes in skin color or temperature; and blisters or necrosis in severe cases. Management includes immediate cessation of drug infusion, assessment and documentation of the site, and aspiration for residual drug if possible. The antidote should be administered if available. The degree of damage may be severe enough to necessitate surgical intervention [53].

Infections

Infections are a major complication associated with central venous ports, particularly in cancer patients due to their immunosuppressed state. Most catheter-related infections arise through two mechanisms: (A) skin infection at the access site, which may involve the subcutaneous pocket and lead to the migration of pathogens along the external catheter surface, and (B) contamination of the catheter hub, resulting in intraluminal colonization and subsequent seeding of pathogens into the bloodstream. It is rare for the infusate to be the source of infection [15].

If the optimal insertion site is selected, experienced operators perform the catheter insertion, strict sterile techniques are adopted, and trained nursing staff provide catheter care, there appears to be no significant difference in infection rates when comparing subclavian, internal jugular, and femoral sites [54]. Complications arising from hematogenous seeding may include endocarditis, suppurative thrombosis, osteomyelitis, and metastatic site infections.

Diagnosis relies on the presence of clinical manifestations of infection, such as fever, swelling at the insertion site, hypotension, chills, and signs of sudden-onset sepsis following infusion. Evidence of catheter colonization can be confirmed through blood cultures and blood samples obtained from a peripheral vein as well as from the central catheter [55].

The treatment of infections is based on targeted antibiotic therapy, guided by the type of bacteria identified, and may necessitate the removal of the catheter. Salvage techniques for the catheter may be considered only under specific conditions: difficulty in replacing the catheter, sterile blood cultures after 48–72 hours, absence of signs of port infection, lack of metastatic complications in cancer patients, presence of a medically treatable pathogen, and hemodynamic stability of the patient [56].

When the catheter is removed, the catheter tip should be cultured rather than the subcutaneous segment. For subcutaneous ports, culture of the material within the port reservoir should also be included, as it is more sensitive than catheter tip cultures. The routine use of intravenous antibiotics prior to catheter insertion has not been shown to reduce the incidence of tunnel or pocket infections and is therefore not recommended [57–59].

Thrombosis

Catheter-related thrombosis (CRT) is a common complication in patients requiring long-term vascular access. In cancer patients, this issue is particularly significant, as they have a five- to seven-fold increased risk of thrombosis [60]. Specific conditions associated with cancer, such as stasis due to immobilization or blood flow obstruction, surgery, infections, endothelial damage from chemotherapeutic agents, and abnormalities in blood coagulation—including specific procoagulant activities of cancer cells, decreased levels of coagulation inhibitors, impaired fibrinolysis, increased antiphospholipid antibodies, activated protein C resistance, enhanced platelet aggregation, and interactions among various coagulation and inflammatory factors—contribute to the hypercoagulable and thrombophilic state observed in these patients [61].

CRT refers to the formation of blood clots on the outer or inner wall of a catheter, leading to mural thrombosis. The incidence of CRT appears to be lower in patients with cancer who have implantable ports compared to those with peripherally inserted central catheters (PICCs) [62]. Regarding the potential role of insertion technique in inducing CRT, ultrasound-guided catheter insertion into a larger vein, which reduces the number of insertion attempts and positions the catheter tip in the largest achievable vein segment, may lower the risk of thrombosis by decreasing compression or friction against the vessel wall [63, 64]. Patient-related factors include sex, advanced age, prolonged immobilization, history of venous thromboembolism (VTE), and either acquired or hereditary states of blood hypercoagulability [65–67].

The rate of CRT is high, ranging from 27% to 66%, but only about one-third of cases become symptomatic. Clinical symptoms may include local pain or a burning sensation during injection, redness, swelling, or edema. In cases where thrombosis is suspected, Doppler ultrasound is the most commonly used diagnostic test due to its availability and noninvasive nature. Venography, CT, or magnetic resonance imaging should be considered if ultrasound results are negative but suspicion of thrombosis persists [68].

CRT can lead to major complications such as pulmonary embolism and sepsis, as well as minor complications including loss of catheter function, fibrin sleeve formation, and superficial thrombophlebitis [69]. When thrombosis occurs, medical treatment and catheter removal are potential options. Thrombolytic therapy may be used in acute cases [70].

In subacute and chronic cases, in the absence of specific contraindications, anticoagulant therapy should be initiated as soon as possible and continued for at least 3 months. The catheter may remain in place if it is still necessary for the patient's condition, provided there is no infection and the thrombosis does not affect the tip while allowing for regular function. Mandatory indications for catheter removal include infected thrombus, malposition of the tip, and irreversible occlusion of the lumen. The risk of embolization during catheter removal has been reported [71].

Low molecular weight heparins remain the most commonly used anticoagulants, particularly for patients with cancer [72], while direct oral anticoagulants represent a potential alternative [73]. Pharmacological prophylaxis is not routinely recommended but should be considered in patients with cancer who have a previous history of thrombosis. Continuing therapy beyond 3 months is advisable if the catheter remains in place or in cases of prior episodes of deep venous thrombosis [60].

References

1. Galloway S, Bodenham A. Long-term central venous access. Br J Anaesth. 2004;92(5):722–34. https://doi.org/10.1093/bja/aeh109. Epub 2004 Mar 5. PMID: 15003979.
2. Möller JC, Reiss I, Schaible T. Vascular access in neonates and infants--indications, routes, techniques and devices, complications. Intensive Care World. 1995;12(2):48–53. PMID: 10150755.
3. Taber SW, Bergamini TM. Long-term venous access: indications and choice of site and catheter. Semin Vasc Surg. 1997;10(3):130–4. PMID: 9304728.
4. Horattas MC, Trupiano J, Hopkins S, Pasini D, Martino C, Murty A. Changing concepts in long-term central venous access: catheter selection and cost savings. Am J Infect Control. 2001;29(1):32–40. https://doi.org/10.1067/mic.2001.111536. PMID: 11172316.
5. Kubiak A, Jazmati T, Sare A, Kumar A, Shukla PA. Overutilization of peripherally inserted central venous catheters in the hospital setting. J Radiol Nurs. 2020;39(4):302–4. ISSN 1546-0843. https://doi.org/10.1016/j.jradnu.2020.06.002.
6. Mikolajczak A, Seburn S, Ward S, Barra MK. 9-190 – Ensuring appropriate Peripherally Inserted Central Catheter (PICC) utilization. Am J Infect Control. 2016;44(6, Supplement):S90. ISSN 0196-6553. https://doi.org/10.1016/j.ajic.2016.04.107.
7. Baskin JL, Pui CH, Reiss U, Wilimas JA, Metzger ML, Ribeiro RC, Howard SC. Management of occlusion and thrombosis associated with long-term indwelling central venous catheters. Lancet. 2009;374(9684):159–69. https://doi.org/10.1016/S0140-6736(09)60220-8. PMID: 19595350; PMCID: PMC2814365.
8. Periard D, Monney P, Waeber G, Zurkinden C, Mazzolai L, Hayoz D, Doenz F, Zanetti G, Wasserfallen JB, Denys A. Randomized controlled trial of peripherally inserted central catheters vs. peripheral catheters for middle duration in-hospital intravenous therapy. J Thromb Haemost. 2008;6(8):1281–8. https://doi.org/10.1111/j.1538-7836.2008.03053.x. Epub 2008 Jun 6. PMID: 18541001.
9. Park S, Moon S, Pai H, Kim B. Appropriate duration of peripherally inserted central catheter maintenance to prevent central line-associated bloodstream infection. PLoS One. 2020;15(6):e0234966. https://doi.org/10.1371/journal.pone.0234966. PMID: 32569313; PMCID: PMC7307762.
10. Woller SC, Stevens SM, Evans RS. The Michigan Appropriateness Guide for Intravenous Catheters (MAGIC) initiative: a summary and review of peripherally inserted central catheter and venous catheter appropriate use. J Hosp Med. 2016;11(4):306–10. https://doi.org/10.1002/jhm.2525. Epub 2015 Dec 14. PMID: 26662622.
11. Lindquester WS, Dhangana R, Warhadpande S, Amesur NB. Effects of the MAGIC guidelines on PICC placement volume: advanced practice provider and physician trends among medicare beneficiaries from 2010 to 2018. AJR Am J Roentgenol. 2021;216(5):1387–91. https://doi.org/10.2214/AJR.20.23704. Epub 2020 Aug 26. PMID: 32845711.
12. DeVries M, Sleweon T. Bridging the gap: introduction of an antimicrobial peripherally inserted central catheter (PICC) in response to high PICC central line-associated bloodstream infection incidence. Br J Nurs. 2021;30(19):S16–22. https://doi.org/10.12968/bjon.2021.30.19.S16. PMID: 34723657.
13. Iida Y, Hongo K, Onoda T, Kita Y, Ishihara Y, Takabayashi N, Kobayashi R, Hiramatsu T. Use of catheter with 2-methacryloyloxyethyl phosphorylcholine polymer coating is associated with long-term availability of central venous port. Sci Rep. 2021;11(1):5385. https://doi.org/10.1038/s41598-021-84885-4. PMID: 33686152; PMCID: PMC7940397.
14. Braun U, Lorenz E, Weimann C, Sturm H, Karimov I, Ettl J, Meier R, Wohlgemuth WA, Berger H, Wildgruber M. Mechanic and surface properties of central-venous port catheters after removal: a comparison of polyurethane and silicon rubber materials. J Mech Behav Biomed Mater. 2016;64:281–91. https://doi.org/10.1016/j.jmbbm.2016.08.002. Epub 2016 Aug 5. PMID: 27552159.
15. McGee DC, Gould MK. Preventing complications of central venous catheterization. N Engl J Med. 2003;348(12):1123–33. https://doi.org/10.1056/NEJMra011883. PMID: 12646670.
16. Safety Committee of Japanese Society of Anesthesiologists. Practical guide for safe central venous catheterization and management 2017. J Anesth. 2020;34(2):167–86. https://doi.org/10.1007/s00540-019-02702-9. Epub 2019 Nov 30. PMID: 31786676; PMCID: PMC7223734.
17. Lim SH, Smith MP, Machin SJ, et al. A prospective randomized study of prophylactic teicoplanin to prevent early Hickman catheter-related sepsis in patients receiving intensive chemotherapy for haematological malignancies. Eur J Haematol Suppl. 1993;54:10–3.
18. Graninger W, Assadian O, Lagler H, et al. The role of glycopeptides in the treatment of intravascular catheterrelated infections. Clin Microbiol Infect. 2002;8:310–5.
19. Centers for Disease Control. Guidelines for the prevention of intravascular catheter-related infections. MMWR Morb Mortal Wkly Rep. 2002;51:1–36.
20. O'Grady NP, Alexander M, Burns LA, Dellinger EP, Garland J, Heard SO, Lipsett PA, Masur H, Mermel LA, Pearson ML, Raad II, Randolph AG, Rupp ME, Saint S, Healthcare Infection Control Practices Advisory Committee. Guidelines for the prevention of intravascular catheter-related infections. Am J Infect Control. 2011;39(4 Suppl 1):S1–34. https://doi.org/10.1016/j.ajic.2011.01.003. PMID: 21511081.
21. Practice guidelines for central venous access 2020: an updated report by the American society of Anesthesiologists Task Force on Central Venous Access. Anesthesiology. 2020;132:8e43.

22. Gebauer B, El-Sheik M, Vogt M, Wagner HJ. Combined ultrasound and fluoroscopy guided port catheter implantation–high success and low complication rate. Eur J Radiol. 2009;69(3):517–22. https://doi.org/10.1016/j.ejrad.2007.10.018. PMID: 19340958.
23. Lamperti M, Bodenham AR, Pittiruti M, Blaivas M, Augoustides JG, Elbarbary M, Pirotte T, Karakitsos D, Ledonne J, Doniger S, Scoppettuolo G, Feller-Kopman D, Schummer W, Biffi R, Desruennes E, Melniker LA, Verghese ST. International evidence-based recommendations on ultrasound-guided vascular access. Intensive Care Med. 2012;38:1105–17.
24. Biffi R, Orsi F, Pozzi S, et al. Best choice of central venous insertion site for the prevention of catheter-related complications in adult patients who need cancer therapy: a randomized trial. Ann Oncol. 2009;20:935–40.
25. Biffi R, Pozzi S, Bonomo G, Della Vigna P, Monfardini L, Radice D, Rotmensz N, Zampino MG, Fazio N, Orsi F. Cost effectiveness of different central venous approaches for port placement and use in adult oncology patients: evidence from a randomized three-arm trial. Ann Surg Oncol. 2014;21(12):3725–31. https://doi.org/10.1245/s10434-014-3784-5. Epub 2014 May 20. PMID: 24841352.
26. Wagner HJ, Teichgräber U, Gebauer B, Kalinowski M. Die transjuguläre Implantation venöser Portkathetersysteme [Transjugular implantation of venous port catheter systems]. Rofo. 2003;175(11):1539–44. German. https://doi.org/10.1055/s-2003-43406. PMID: 14610706.
27. Manudeep AR, Manjula BP, Dinesh Kumar US. Comparison of peres' formula and radiological landmark formula for optimal depth of insertion of right internal jugular venous catheters. Indian J Crit Care Med. 2020;24(7):527–30. https://doi.org/10.5005/jp journals-10071-23478. PMID. 32963434; PMCID: PMC7482340.
28. Zakhour R, Chaftari AM, Raad II. Catheter-related infections in patients with haematological malignancies: novel preventive and therapeutic strategies. Lancet Infect Dis. 2016;16(11):e241–50.
29. Moss JG, Wu O, Bodenham AR, Agarwal R, Menne TF, Jones BL, et al. Central venous access devices for the delivery of systemic anticancer therapy (CAVA): a randomised controlled trial. Lancet. 2021;398:403–15.
30. Sznajder JI, Zveibil FR, Bitterman H, Weiner P, Bursztein S. Central vein catheterization. Failure and complication rates by three percutaneous approaches. Arch Intern Med. 1986;146(2):259–61. https://doi.org/10.1001/archinte.146.2.259. PMID: 3947185.
31. Lucey B, Varghese JC, Haslam P, Lee MJ. Routine chest radiographs after central line insertion: mandatory postprocedural evaluation or unnecessary waste of resources? Cardiovasc Intervent Radiol. 1999;22:381–4.
32. Lanza C, Russo M, Fabrizzi G. Central venous cannulation: are routine chest radiographs necessary after B-mode and colour Doppler sonography check? Pediatr Radiol. 2006;36:1252–6.
33. Giacomini M, Iapichino G, Armani S, et al. How to avoid and manage a pneumothorax. J Vasc Access. 2006;7:7–14.
34. Ellis LM, Vogel SB, Copeland EM III. Central venous catheter vascular erosions. Diagnosis and clinical course. Ann Surg. 1989;209:475–8.
35. Guilbert MC, Elkouri S, Bracco D, et al. Arterial trauma during central venous catheter insertion: case series, review and proposed algorithm. J Vasc Surg. 2008;48:918–25; discussion 925.
36. Biswas S, Sidani M, Abrol S. Emergent median sternotomy for mediastinal hematoma: a rare omplication following internal jugular vein catheterization for chemoport insertion—a case report and review of relevant literature. Case Rep Anesthesiol. 2014;2014:190172.
37. Wang L, Jia L, Jiang A. Pathology of catheter-related complications: what we need to know and what should be discovered. J Int Med Res. 2022;50(10):3000605221127890. https://doi.org/10.1177/03000605221127890. PMID: 36268763; PMCID: PMC9597033.
38. Crain MR, Horton MG, Mewissen MW. Fibrin sheaths complicating central venous catheters. AJR Am J Roentgenol. 1998;171(2):341–6. https://doi.org/10.2214/ajr.171.2.9694448. PMID: 9694448.
39. Santilli J. Fibrin sheaths and central venous catheter occlusions: diagnosis and management. Tech Vasc Interv Radiol. 2002;5(2):89–94. https://doi.org/10.1053/tvir.2002.36048. PMID: 12489047.
40. Hinke DH, Zandt-Stastny DA, Goodman LR, Quebbeman EJ, Krzywda EA, Andris DA. Pinch-off syndrome: a complication of implantable subclavian venous access devices. Radiology. 1990;177(2):353–6. https://doi.org/10.1148/radiology.177.2.2217768. PMID: 2217768.
41. Chuah JS, Wong WL, Bakin S, Lim RZM, Lee EP, Tan JH. Pinch-off syndrome from a chemoport catheter successfully managed with endovascular retrieval. Ann Med Surg (Lond). 2021;65:102294. https://doi.org/10.1016/j.amsu.2021.102294. PMID: 33948169; PMCID: PMC8079954.
42. Aitken DR, Minton JP. The "pinch-off sign": a warning of impending problems with permanent subclavian catheters. Am J Surg. 1984;148(5):633–6. https://doi.org/10.1016/0002-9610(84)90340-4. PMID: 6496853.
43. Bessoud B, de Baere T, Kuoch V, Desruennes E, Cosset MF, Lassau N, Roche A. Experience at a single institution with endovascular treatment of mechanical complications caused by implanted central venous access devices in pediatric and adult patients. AJR Am J Roentgenol. 2003;180(2):527–32. https://doi.org/10.2214/ajr.180.2.1800527. PMID: 12540466.
44. Harrison E, Lal S. Central venous catheter embolisation. BMJ Case Rep. 2012;2012:bcr2012007249. https://doi.org/10.1136/bcr-2012-007249. PMID: 23175013; PMCID: PMC4544544.

45. Winston CB, Wechsler RJ, Kane M. Vertebral vein migration of a long-term central venous access catheter: a cause of brachial plexopathy. J Thorac Imaging. 1994;9(2):98–100. https://doi.org/10.1097/00005382-199421000-00008. PMID: 8207788.
46. Mahon T, Lawrence D Sr. Technical report: an injection technique for repositioning subclavian catheters. Clin Radiol. 1991;44:197–8.
47. Roizental M, Hartnell GG. The misplaced central venous catheter: a long loop technique for repositioning. J Vasc Interv Radiol. 1995;6:263–5.
48. Gordon Hartnell G, Gates J, Suojanen JN, Clouse ME. Transfemoral repositioning of malpositioned central venous catheters. Cardiovasc Intervent Radiol. 1996;19(5):329–31. https://doi.org/10.1007/bf02570184.
49. Kassner E. Evaluation and treatment of chemotherapy extravasation injuries. J Pediatr Oncol Nurs. 2000;17(3):135–48. https://doi.org/10.1053/jpon.2000.8063. PMID: 10944862.
50. Gallieni M, Pittiruti M, Biffi R. Vascular access in oncology patients. CA Cancer J Clin. 2008;58(6):323–46. https://doi.org/10.3322/CA.2008.0015. Epub 2008 Oct 29. PMID: 18971486.
51. Bozkurt AK, Uzel B, Akman C, et al. Intrathoracic extravasation of antineoplastic agents: case report and systematic review. Am J Clin Oncol. 2003;26:121–3.
52. Pham TD, Tsunoyama T. Exploring extravasation in cancer patients. Cancers (Basel). 2024;16(13):2308. https://doi.org/10.3390/cancers16132308. PMID: 39001371; PMCID: PMC11240416.
53. Deshpande KS, Hatem C, Ulrich HL, et al. The incidence of infectious complications of central venous catheters at the subclavian, internal jugular, and femoral sites in an intensive care unit population. Crit Care Med. 2005;33:13–20.
54. Bouza E, Burillo A, Muñoz P. Catheter-related infections: diagnosis and intravascular treatment. Clin Microbiol Infect. 2002;8(5):265–74. https://doi.org/10.1046/j.1469-0691.2002.00385.x. PMID: 12047403.
55. Schiffer CA, Mangu PB, Wade JC, et al. Central venous catheter care for the patient with cancer: American Society of Clinical Oncology clinical practice guideline. J Clin Oncol. 2013;31(10):1357–70.
56. van de Wetering MD, van Woensel JB. Prophylactic antibiotics for preventing early central venous catheter Grampositive infections in oncology patients. Cochrane Database Syst Rev. 2007;1(1):CD003295.
57. Covey AM, Toro-Pape FW, Thornton RH, et al. Totally implantable venous access device placement by interventional radiologists: are prophylactic antibiotics necessary? J Vasc Interv Radiol. 2012;23(3):358–62.
58. Agnelli G, Verso M. Management of venous thromboembolism in patients with cancer. J Thromb Haemost. 2011;9(Suppl 1):316–24.
59. Gouin-Thibault I, Achkar A, Samama MM. The thrombophilic state in cancer patients. Acta Haematol. 2001;106(1–2):33–42. https://doi.org/10.1159/000046587. PMID: 11549775.
60. Girardi L, Di Nisio M, Candeloro M, Valeriani E, Ageno W. Catheter-related deep vein thrombosis: where are we at and where are we going? Updates and ongoing unmet clinical needs. Eur J Clin Investig. 2024:e14311. https://doi.org/10.1111/eci.14311. Epub ahead of print. PMID: 39262322.
61. Brewer C. Reducing upper extremity deep vein thrombosis when inserting PICCs. Br J Nurs. 2012;21(14):S12–7. https://doi.org/10.12968/BJON.2012.21.SUP14.S12.
62. Orme RMLE, McSwiney MM, Chamberlain-Webber RFO. Fatal cardiac tamponade as a result of a peripherally inserted central venous catheter: a case report and review of the literature. Br J Anaesth. 2007;99(3):384–8. https://doi.org/10.1093/BJA/AEM181.
63. Chopra V, et al. Risk of venous thromboembolism associated with peripherally inserted central catheters: a systematic review and meta-analysis. Lancet. 2013;382(9889):311–25.
64. Lowell JA, Bothe A Jr. Central venous catheter-related thrombosis. Surg Oncol Clin N Am. 1995;4:479–92.
65. Tran BH, Nguyen TJ, Hwang BH, et al. Risk factors associated with venous thromboembolism in 49,028 mastectomy patients. Breast. 2013;22:444–8.
66. Baskin JL, Pui CH, Reiss U, et al. Management of occlusion and thrombosis associated with long-term indwelling central venous catheters. Lancet. 2009;374:159–69.
67. Lee AY, Kamphuisen PW. Epidemiology and prevention of catheter-related thrombosis in patients with cancer. J Thromb Haemost. 2012;10:1491–9.
68. Rodenhuis S, van't Hek LG, Vlasveld LT, Kröger R, Dubbelman R, van Tol RG. Central venous catheter associated thrombosis of major veins: thrombolytic treatment with recombinant tissue plasminogen activator. Thorax. 1993;48(5):558–9. https://doi.org/10.1136/thx.48.5.558. PMID: 8322245; PMCID: PMC464517.
69. Zuha R, Price T, Powles R, Treleaven J. Paradoxical emboli after central venous catheter removal. Ann Oncol. 2000;11:885–6.
70. Farge D, Frere C, Connors JM, et al. 2022 international clinical practice guidelines for the treatment and prophylaxis of venous thromboembolism in patients with cancer, including patients with COVID-19. Lancet Oncol. 2022;23(7):e334–47. https://doi.org/10.1016/S1470-2045(22)00160-7.
71. Valeriani E, Di Nisio M, Porceddu E, et al. Anticoagulant treatment for upper extremity deep vein thrombosis: a systematic review and meta-analysis. J Thromb Haemost. 2022;20(3):661–70. https://doi.org/10.1111/JTH.15614.
72. Key NS, Khorana AA, Kuderer NM, et al. Venous thromboembolism prophylaxis and treatment in patients with cancer: ASCO clinical practice guideline update. J Clin Oncol. 2020;38(5):496-520. https://doi.org/10.1200/JCO.19.01461.
73. Schrag D, Uno H, Rosovsky R, et al. Direct Oral Anticoagulants vs Low-Molecular-Weight Heparin and Recurrent VTE in Patients With Cancer: A Randomized Clinical Trial. JAMA. 2023;329(22):1924–33. https://doi.org/10.1001/jama.2023.7843.

Special Considerations 7

Lorenzo Monfardini

Central Venous Cannulation in Patients with Coagulopathy or Anticoagulation

Coagulopathy can be such a condition frequently recurring in clinical daily practice. It can be a consequence of a medical condition (liver failure, sepsis, trauma) or can be induced by medical treatments [1]. In both cases, the first measure is his correction [2] but not always can be as easily and promptly achieved.

Anticoagulation or antiplatelet therapy following vascular devices implantation has significantly impacted on invasive percutaneous procedures. In such a scenario since the coagulation or the aggregation mitigation has a therapeutic intent, the treatment removal should be carefully evaluated depending on pros and cons. Among several guidelines on such topic, the most complete and easily consultable are provided by the Society of Interventional Radiology: the different medications with regard to antiplatelet or anticoagulant mechanism of action are analyzed [3] and clinical considerations are provided [4]. According to this approach, the most important consideration for central venous access is represented by their classification within procedures with a low bleeding risk. More in detail, the simple venipuncture without subcutaneous tunnel creation requires PT/INR and platelet count but can be safely performed:

- Correcting INR to within the range of ≤1.5–1.8
- Transfuse platelet only if $<50 \times 10^9/L$

Therefore, the conditions in which single or dual antiplatelet or anticoagulation therapy should be corrected are strictly limited. The most relevant technical factor, however, which has been worldwide endorsed to ultimately confirm this approach is ultrasound (US) guidance. Later than a decade, the first retrospective experiences opting out the need for coagulation correction in central venous access with US guidance were available in cancer patients with hemostatic disorders [5]. Since then, the agreement on such theme has been undisputed [6, 7] and recent meta-analysis does not even suggest correction for INR higher of 1.8 and/or platelet count below $50 \times 10^9/L$ [8]. The reason itself is very obvious indeed being US a useful tool for seeing what is normally not noticeable with the blind technique. However, the most important factor for a proper use of US guidance remains an appropriate training in basic diagnostic US. Managing properly even the slightest anatomical detail allows to a deep understanding of what vessel should be avoided before reaching the planned target [9].

L. Monfardini (✉)
Interventional Radiology San Giuseppe Hospital, Multimedica Group IRCCS, Milan, Italy
e-mail: lorenzo.monfardini@multimedica.it

R. Lanocita, M. Lamperti (eds.), *Practical Guide to Central Venous Cannulation*,
https://doi.org/10.1007/978-3-031-90326-7_7

For jugular and subclavian cannulation, the cause of hematoma during the learning curve of US-guided approach is not the direct puncture of the correspondent artery itself, but more often small branches of the thyrocervical artery or the inferior thyroideal artery (Fig. 7.1). For this reason, it is possible to speculate that catheter placed by interventional radiologists has been excluded by recent and robust evidence of US guidance usefulness [10]. Those details are indeed of paramount importance in patients with platelet or coagulation failure. Further technical details that could be considered affecting bleeding risk in vein cannulation are needle size and number of cannulation attempts: if more than one needle pass has been described in association with increased bleeding risk, the same evidence for big needle caliper is lacking [8]. In fact, this last review lists 22 retrospective studies for central vein cannulation in coagulopathic patients with a needle size ranging from 18 to 22 gauge without significant difference in complications. However once again, borrowing interventional radiologist's techniques could help: micropuncture technique (22 G needle plus 0.018 inch guide wire) has been successfully described as the only way to cannulate bile ducts or renal pelvis in a poor distension condition [11]. A similar condition could be faced with a collapsing central vein in case of dehydration or low central venous pressure. Yet the reduced stiffness and the higher banding attitude of a 22 G needle imply a great operator confidence with such tool.

From a practical point of view, the correct approach for a central venous line placement in a patient with coagulation or platelet deficiency should imply medical correction or treatment suspension as the last chance. The following suggestions can be considered for a safe outcome:

1. Coagulation assessment and platelet count.
2. US examination for the different site examination: since there is not a clear evidence about which is the safest vein, the final choice is left to the operator's confidence.

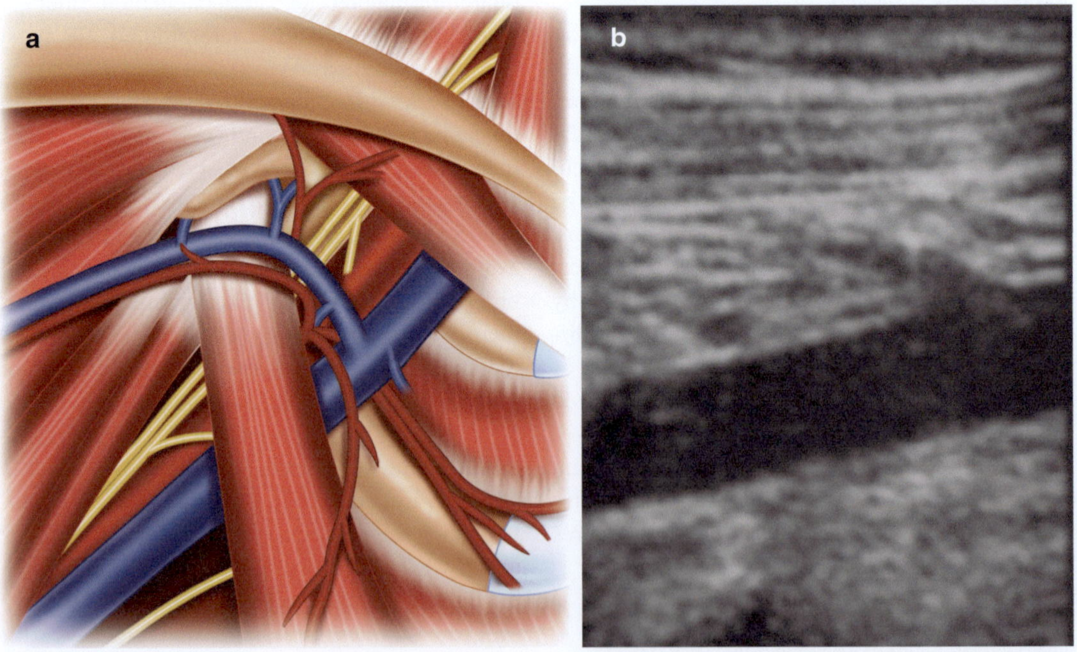

Fig. 7.1 The table of the vascular anatomy in the subclavian region (**a**) and the correspondent ultrasound image (**b**): the thyrocervical trunk and its main branches are the main accountable for the corresponding arterial supply. A blind approach of the subclavian vein with an arterial undesired hematoma is most likely the consequence of crossing those smaller vessels rather than a direct subclavian artery puncture

3. Correct use of US guidance preferably with long-axis technique to achieve a precise real time monitoring of the needle tip position.
4. In case of difficult anatomical location or "squeezed veins," consider micropuncture technique.
5. Perform a final ultrasound check at the end of the procedure to exclude any possible hematomas.
6. Plan a bedside control of venipuncture site to report oozing or late onset hematomas. Such measure should be lasted as long as coagulation is compromised.

In conclusion, recalling the opening theme of risk/benefit balance is possible to argue that central venous cannulation in coagulopathy, especially when performed with in plane US guidance, is worth the poor risk of hematoma.

Complications of Central Venous Cannulation: Air Embolism and Cardiac Perforation

In one of the largest prospective multicentric studies including more than 12,000 central venous catheter insertions, minor mechanical complications occurred in 8% of insertions and major complications in less than 1% [12]. The main background disclosed in the title is however the intent to collect data "in the US-guided era." Such a statement clearly defines the author's attitude to consider central vein cannulation a safe procedure for trained operators. Among major complications in fact, only arterial catheterization and pneumothorax are listed as relevant and none of the causes of death were related with the procedure. But a more recent prospective single institution study [13], while recognizing major immediate insertion-related complications not directly responsible for any death, showed an association with increased 30-day, 90-day, and 180-day mortality. This was mainly explained because major immediate insertion-related complications can delay treatment or require invasive interventions, which in turn could affect mortality. In summary, giving ultrasound guidance for granted, both the cited studies indicate risk stratification as the most useful tool to prevent complications; notably high body mass index, operator limited experience and male gender require special attention.

Different situations deserve specific mention because of their anecdotal incidence:

1. *Air embolism* has recently gained prominence during the last decade in the interventional radiologist's practice because of lung biopsies. The direct communication between lung small veins and the corrispondent bronchial branch could eventually lead to an air leak in the systemic circulation in some circumstances such as small nodules, cough during procedures, or prone positioning. Even if notably rare such condition is potentially death-related (Fig. 7.2) and a lot of debate has been made on such topic [14] without a clear evidence about how much the recalled risk factors really influence air embolism incidence. All authors however do agree about how impactful can be such complication consequences not just for the patient but in second instance even for the operator. Vein catheterization itself can lead even more rarely to a systemic air embolism because of lung filter. This is the reason why only few case reports are available and only a single

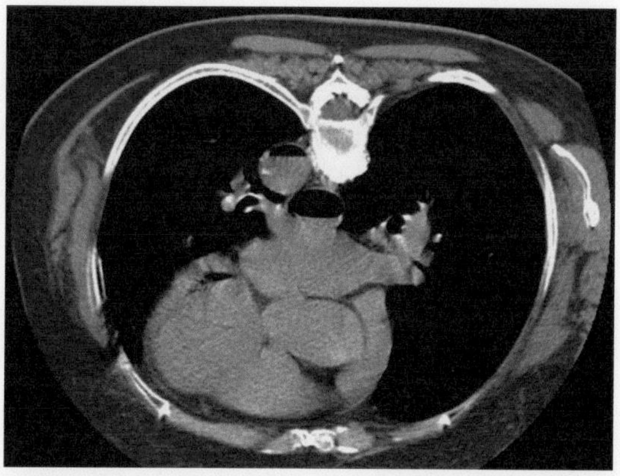

Fig. 7.2 A case of massive air embolism after a lung biopsy: a notable amount of air is trapped in the thoracic aorta as well as in the right coronary artery. Consequences with such a scenario could be life-threatening

review collecting much of the available literature is mainly focused on cerebral air embolism [15]. However, interesting speculations are provided that can be of interest to clinicians dealing with central venous lines. Firstly, according to other published experiences, the cannulation itself has been founded in association with air embolism in less than 10% of cases. Most of air embolism cases described are related with central venous line removal, maintenance, or substitution [16]. Secondly, the cases in which cardiac shunt was investigated were the minority, but only in less than the half, a real cardiac or intrapulmonary shunt was evident. For the remanent cases, the mechanism that could more probably be the cause of brain suffering is retrograde venous embolism, but this is just a speculation since even with CT scan, it is actually difficult to identify the precise site of the smallest bubble. Lastly, this paper was focused only on neurological consequences excluding cardiac embolism which consequences could even lead to a worst case scenario. Leaving the speculations behind, once again some practical advices can be more useful in order to avoid air embolism in the first instance at least in the venous system:

- During cannulation especially with larger needles (18 gauge or more), always consider a syringe connected with the needle and the catheter itself both filled with saline.
- For larger devices (plasmapheresis and dialysis), pay attention during percutaneous dilatation while removing large diameter dilators. Digital pressure on the puncture site is useful to stabilize the guidewire but mostly to avoid bleeding or hematomas. Moreover, bleeding out means no air leaking in.
- For large catheter needing peel away introducing system, pay special attention. Even peel away system for central venous port sizing up from 7 F can be large enough to allow a substantial amount of air to be collected in the right atrium in a short time. If the switch from guide and dilator to the catheter is not made with a proper timing and during an inspiration, air will most likely be aspired in the central venous system. A simple time matching Valsalva maneuver is protective.
- As previously discussed, the most frequent circumstance associated with central line air embolism is its bed-care. For this reason, only adequately trained operators should manage central lines being aware of adequately applying manual pressure on the puncture site when removing or substituting catheters. In case of dyspnea, cough, and drop of saturation, Trendelenburg position and oxygen mask supplementation are usually sufficient to successfully solve the situation since the air is adsorbed by alveoli and expelled.
- If air embolism reach lung filter symptoms, severity usually depends on the amount of air leaked and the distance from the venipuncture site to right atrium: femoral and peripheral approaches are less likely to induce lung symptomatic air embolism. The external air mixture coming not by airways but by capillaries usually stimulates vasoconstriction that induce a transient reduction of oxygen saturation levels, dyspnea, and cough.
- In the sporadic occurrence of embolism extended to systemic circulation, symptoms may change depending on the anatomical location of the leaked air. Intracranial and coronary distribution provide stroke and acute infarction like signs, respectively. In this case, Trendelenburg and oxygen are useful to limit the damage but are not of therapeutic value. A CT scan should be immediately performed keeping a stable decubitus to demonstrate air in the suspected anatomical site. Anesthesiologist supervision is mandatory.

2. *Cardiac tamponade* is another occurrence reported sporadically. A single review is available [17] collecting few reports of one to two cases each, not even collected in a proper table. The main issue is described as the perpetual continued traumatic effect of rigid

catheters (polyurethane) on the cardiac wall as the main chronic cause. To find out a description of acute cardiac tamponade during the line placement is even more difficult. Such event has been solved at the root once again by interventional radiologists with the continuous fluoroscopic monitoring. However for a bedside procedure, a simple chest X-ray should be always performed right to exclude any conflict with the cardiac wall and the catheter. The ideal point for the catheter tip has been described since two decades [18] at the Rx projective junction of superior vena cava and right atrium. Once again from a practical point of view, following such easy rule should be reasonably protective from such an occurrence. Moreover, the time required for a chronical cardiac wall damage induced by a temporary central line decubitus is longer than the normal supposed on site time before its removal. Therefore, this kind of problem should be only considered for long permanence totally implantable devices; the need for repositioning the catheter in such a scenario has in fact been described once again, since more than two decades [19]. This is the main reason why a perioperative fluoroscopy setting is highly recommended.

Management of Difficult or Failed Central Venous Access

The definition of a "difficult central venous access" is strictly bonded to failure. Practically speaking, a difficult central cannulation occurs when the catheter cannot be entered into the vein in one attempt after one or more failure. Nurses literature has several definitions and descriptions of difficult access [20, 21] which in all cases are solved with US guidance. Moreover, a deep arguing is available for peripheral difficult access [22] but not for central lines. For physician even trained in central venous lines, the problem is more complex. All the technical suggestions listed in the previous and following chapters are useful while facing difficult central venous lines; however, the real deal for which medical doctors should be trained is how far to push the indication for a central venous line in difficult cases. In fact, if for any emergency scenario there is no doubt about having a central venous line "whatever it takes," in different cases, a risk-benefit analysis is the most appropriate way to deal with the single case. From the purely technical perspective, a venous access is always achievable: interventional radiologist dealing with devices placed in every part of the body via whatever percutaneous approach would find a way to gain a venous access even in the most difficult situations [23]. The choice of a "guidance technique upgrade" trough fluoroscopy reaching computed tomography allows to cannulate even deeper central veins. However to decide if the risk is worth the benefit should always be decided in a multidisciplinary background in order to carefully weight pros and cons.

All the different explanations for a supposed or real challenging access may depend on clinical, anatomical, and technical details, and their full analysis could be excessive. However, some practical advice depending on the different difficult cannulation scenarios could be helpful:

- BMI is a measure of body fat based on the height and weight of the individual. A significative variation in subcutaneous thickness may represent a challenge in obtaining venous access even with US guidance. A prior evaluation of anatomy for obese patient is helpful to really understand how deep the venipuncture is supposed to happen. If the normal linear probe is not enough to clearly visualize the vessel, consider to change with a convex one. Once again, such an adjustment requires a higher level of confidence with US technique. Another parameter deserving attention is needle length: even if it may seem more than obvious, the large majority of central cannulation sets include needle not longer than 7 or 8 cm, measures not useful for obese patients. Lastly, dilation of guidewire path should be careful for the risk of its bending in the soft fat layer. If for patients with medium to mild subcutaneous layer US visualization is not compromised, some issue could be faced in patients with relevant reduction of subcutaneous layers such as cachectic patients. The lack of useful layers can turn US evaluation of needle path in a real challenge for non-trained operators; especially jugular approach can test even the most skilled interventional radiologists because of the lack of a reliable skin plan to trust for a confident imaging. The sternal extremity of the clavicular bone is indeed a relevant obstacle for a comfortable probe placement especially for skinniest patients. An appropriate amount of sterile gel for a continuous US conduction could help to overcome such issue.

- Clinical factors affecting central line placement could be of different origin. Age itself would deserve a separate discussion. In fact, a med search using as keywords "difficult central venous access" provide almost entirely pediatric publications. In such a setting, the smaller dimension is playing a pivotal role and dedicated physicians already are skilled sonographers. Coagulation defects are already been discussed. Among pathological vein conditions, thrombosis with or without phlebitis is the most commonly affecting central line insertion. Such a situation can be easily detected with US if in the site of insertion but can cause a lot of problems if deeper. After the venipuncture, the guidewire will not advance in the expected position and the result will be a final misplacement or a difficult fluoroscopic negotiation of the guidewire position. In both cases, the only way is to rely on a previous CT scan clarifying the deeper central vein situation. To let a venous line in place in case of thrombosis could only lead to a worse scenario, so the best solution is to choose a different vein approach. Moreover, having a previous CT scan can also be helpful for the anatomical variation detection. Double superior cava vein conditions are not so infrequent and can modify the projective tip position without catheter malfunctioning.
- Technical issues causing a difficult venous access can be defined as the circumstances under which a lack of technology, devices, or skill hampers a safe and effective cannulation. The most important take-home message for such a situation is very simple but not often practiced: refer the patient to a more equipped place of care.

In summary, a reliable venous access can be achieved in the majority of cases, thanks to different imaging techniques as guidance, but pros and cons should be carefully evaluated possibly in a multidisciplinary scenario.

References

1. Giustozzi M, Ehrlinder H, Bongiovanni D, Borovac JA, Guerreiro RA, Gąsecka A, Papakonstantinou PE, Parker WAE. Coagulopathy and sepsis: pathophysiology, clinical manifestations and treatment. Blood Rev. 2021;50:100864. https://doi.org/10.1016/j.blre.2021.100864. Epub 2021 Jun 25. PMID: 34217531.
2. Wallisch WJ, Kidd B, Shen L, Hammer R, Siscel J. Coagulopathy and emergent reversal of anticoagulation. Anesthesiol Clin. 2023;41(1):249–61. https://doi.org/10.1016/j.anclin.2022.10.006. PMID: 36872002.
3. Davidson JC, Rahim S, Hanks SE, Patel IJ, Tam AL, Walker TG, Weinberg I, Wilkins LR, Sarode R. Society of Interventional Radiology Consensus Guidelines for the Periprocedural Management of Thrombotic and Bleeding Risk in Patients Undergoing Percutaneous Image-Guided Interventions-Part I: Review of Anticoagulation Agents and Clinical Considerations: Endorsed by the Canadian Association for Interventional Radiology and the Cardiovascular and Interventional Radiological Society of Europe. J Vasc Interv Radiol. 2019;30(8):1155–67. https://doi.org/10.1016/j.jvir.2019.04.016. Epub 2019 Jun 20. PMID: 31229332.
4. Patel IJ, Rahim S, Davidson JC, Hanks SE, Tam AL, Walker TG, Wilkins LR, Sarode R, Weinberg I. Society of Interventional Radiology Consensus Guidelines for the Periprocedural Management of Thrombotic and Bleeding Risk in Patients Undergoing Percutaneous Image-Guided Interventions-Part II: Recommendations: Endorsed by the Canadian Association for Interventional Radiology and the Cardiovascular and Interventional Radiological Society of Europe. J Vasc Interv Radiol. 2019;30(8):1168–1184.e1. https://doi.org/10.1016/j.jvir.2019.04.017. Epub 2019 Jun 20. PMID: 31229333.

5. Della Vigna P, Monfardini L, Bonomo G, Curigliano G, Agazzi A, Bellomi M, Orsi F. Coagulation disorders in patients with cancer: nontunneled central venous catheter placement with US guidance--a single-institution retrospective analysis. Radiology. 2009;253(1):249–52. https://doi.org/10.1148/radiol.2531081963. Epub 2009 Jun 30. PMID: 19567651.
6. Tercan F, Ozkan U, Oguzkurt L. US-guided placement of central vein catheters in patients with disorders of hemostasis. Eur J Radiol. 2008;65(2):253–6. https://doi.org/10.1016/j.ejrad.2007.04.002. Epub 2007 May 4. PMID: 17482407.
7. Reusz G, Langer C, Hevessy T, Csomós Á. Ultrasound-guided central venous access in patients with uncorrected coagulopathy. Orv Hetil. 2015;156(27):1085–90. https://doi.org/10.1556/650.2015.30194. PMID: 26122903. Hungarian.
8. van de Weerdt EK, Biemond BJ, Baake B, Vermin B, Binnekade JM, van Lienden KP, Vlaar APJ. Central venous catheter placement in coagulopathic patients: risk factors and incidence of bleeding complications. Transfusion. 2017;57:2512–25. https://doi.org/10.1111/trf.14248.
9. Saugel B, Scheeren TWL, Teboul JL. Ultrasound-guided central venous catheter placement: a structured review and recommendations for clinical practice. Crit Care. 2017;21(1):225. https://doi.org/10.1186/s13054-017-1814-y. PMID: 28844205; PMCID: PMC5572160.
10. Teja B, Bosch NA, Diep C, Pereira TV, Mauricio P, Sklar MC, Sankar A, Wijeysundera HC, Saskin R, Walkey A, Wijeysundera DN, Wunsch H. Complication rates of central venous catheters: a systematic review and meta-analysis. JAMA Intern Med. 2024;184(5):474–82. https://doi.org/10.1001/jamainternmed.2023.8232. PMID: 38436976.
11. Pedersoli F, Schröder A, Zimmermann M, et al. Percutaneous transhepatic biliary drainage (PTBD) in patients with dilated vs. nondilated bile ducts: technical considerations and complications. Eur Radiol. 2021;31:3035–41. https://doi.org/10.1007/s00330-020-07368-6.
12. Adrian M, Borgquist O, Kröger T, Linné E, Bentzer P, Spångfors M, Åkeson J, Holmström A, Linnér R, Kander T. Mechanical complications after central venous catheterisation in the ultrasound-guided era: a prospective multicentre cohort study. Br J Anaesth. 2022;129(6):843–50. https://doi.org/10.1016/j.bja.2022.08.036. Epub 2022 Oct 22. PMID: 36280461.
13. Ingefors S, Adrian M, Heckley G, Borgquist O, Kander T. Major immediate insertion-related complications after central venous catheterisation and associations with mortality, length of hospital stay, and costs: a prospective observational study. J Vasc Access. 2025;26:487–96. https://doi.org/10.1177/11297298231222929. Epub ahead of print. PMID: 38267828.
14. Cousin F. Reply to "Percutaneous lung biopsy: smart positioning – prone should be forbidden". Cardiovasc Intervent Radiol. 2020;43(6):940–1. https://doi.org/10.1007/s00270-020-02435-3. Epub 2020 Feb 24. PMID: 32095841.
15. Pinho J, Amorim JM, Araújo JM, Vilaça H, Ribeiro M, Pereira J, Ferreira C. Cerebral gas embolism associated with central venous catheter: systematic review. J Neurol Sci. 2016;362:160–4. https://doi.org/10.1016/j.jns.2016.01.043. Epub 2016 Jan 22. PMID: 26944140.
16. Brouns R, De Surgeloose D, Neetens I, De Deyn PP. Fatal venous cerebral air embolism secondary to a disconnected central venous catheter. Cerebrovasc Dis. 2006;21(3):212–4. https://doi.org/10.1159/000090795. Epub 2006 Jan 9. PMID: 16401887.
17. Messina Alvarez AA, Bilal MA, Manasrah N, Chaudhary A. Iatrogenic cardiac tamponade secondary to central venous catheter placement: a literature review. Cureus. 2023;15(4):e37695. https://doi.org/10.7759/cureus.37695. PMID: 37206520; PMCID: PMC10191201.
18. Fletcher SJ, Bodenham AR. Safe placement of central venous catheters: where should the tip of the catheter lie? Br J Anaesth. 2000;85(2):188–91. https://doi.org/10.1093/bja/85.2.188. PMID: 10992821.
19. Kincaid EH, Davis PW, Chang MC, Fenstermaker JM, Pennell TC. "Blind" placement of long-term central venous access devices: report of 589 consecutive procedures. Am Surg. 1999;65(6):520–3; discussion 523–4. PMID: 10366205.
20. Sou V, McManus C, Mifflin N, Frost SA, Ale J, Alexandrou E. A clinical pathway for the management of difficult venous access. BMC Nurs. 2017;16:64. https://doi.org/10.1186/s12912-017-0261-z. PMID: 29176933; PMCID: PMC5693534.
21. Armenteros-Yeguas V, Gárate-Echenique L, Tomás-López MA, Cristóbal-Domínguez E, Moreno-de Gusmão B, Miranda-Serrano E, Moraza-Dulanto MI. Prevalence of difficult venous access and associated risk factors in highly complex hospitalised patients. J Clin Nurs. 2017;26(23–24):4267–75. https://doi.org/10.1111/jocn.13750. Epub 2017 Mar 28. PMID: 28165645; PMCID: PMC6084302.
22. Eren H. Difficult intravenous access and its management [Internet]. In: Ultimate guide to outpatient care. IntechOpen; 2022. Available from: https://doi.org/10.5772/intechopen.96613.
23. Smith TP, Ryan JM, Reddan DN. Transhepatic catheter access for hemodialysis. Radiology. 2004;232:246–51. https://doi.org/10.4103/joacp.joacp_329_21. Epub 2022 Feb 21.

Alternative Access Techniques

8

Davide Vailati, Giuseppe Capozzoli, Jacopo Crippa, and Salvatore Barbaro

Percutaneous and Open Surgical Approaches to Central Ventral Access

The surgical approach to central venous catheter (CVC) placement is becoming less common due to advances in radiologic and anaesthesiologic techniques. The need for a high flow rate, long-term therapies, or poor peripheral vein status usually drives the decision to use a central lumen catheterisation. An open surgical approach remains a standard alternative procedure for paediatric patients. An open surgical approach may be considered in adults when a percutaneous approach cannot be achieved or when placing a long-term tunnelled catheter. Typically, totally implanted vascular devices are positioned surgically, and tunnelled CVCs are associated with fewer chronic complications [1]. The surgical approach can be helpful in cases of previous catheter placement, venous access complications, or deep venous thrombosis, limiting the choice of a peripheral approach.

Approaches differ according to the site and respective anatomy. Common sites for surgical (and non-surgical) CVC placement include the following:

- Internal jugular vein
- Subclavian/axillary vein
- Brachial and cephalic vein
- Femoral vein

Choosing one site over another may be challenging and should be based on operator experience, local site conditions, and availability. The preferred site remains controversial. The internal jugular vein is the most common site for temporary CVCs, with strong recommendations for its use in this setting [2]. Subclavian access has been reported as a favourable site for preventing vascular catheter (VC) infection colonisation, although it remains anatomically challenging and difficult to control in case of catheter misplacement [3, 4]. Generally, the access site should be chosen based on local expertise, clinical judgment, and distance from contaminated sites, and in adult patients, the upper body is preferable over the lower body [5].

Ultrasound identification of the vessel is the gold standard in percutaneous CVC placement and is recommended by multiple society guidelines [6]. When an ultrasound approach is

D. Vailati (✉)
Anesthesia and ICU Melegnano Hospital – ASST Melegnano e Martesana, Milan, Italy
e-mail: davide.vailati@asst-melegnano-martesana.it

G. Capozzoli
Anesthesia and ICU Bolzano Hospital, Bozen, Italy

J. Crippa · S. Barbaro
Surgery Department Melegnano Hospital – ASST Melegnano e Martesana, Milan, Italy
e-mail: jacopo.crippa@asst-melegnano-martesana.it; salvatore.barbaro@asst-melegnano-martesana.it

R. Lanocita, M. Lamperti (eds.), *Practical Guide to Central Venous Cannulation*,
https://doi.org/10.1007/978-3-031-90326-7_8

impossible, anatomical landmarks become essential to locate the access site.

The surgical open approach follows similar steps to percutaneous or radiological approaches: catheter selection, access site selection, proper patient positioning, sterile technique, antiseptic procedures, local anaesthesia or sedation, catheter placement, and positioning control. In the case of an open surgical approach, the vein is isolated under direct vision, and a venotomy is performed. The surgical approach is associated with high morbidity, making it not the first choice for adult CVC placement. Common complications include catheter misplacement, bleeding, and infection of the surgical site. If the CVC is not in the correct position, venous thrombosis, bleeding, arrhythmia, and other complications may occur [7]. Specific guidelines on the length of the catheter to be inserted have been published [1], along with other ECG-guided techniques [8], to minimize the risk of VC misplacement.

Anatomical Landmarks

The internal jugular vein is one of the most utilised accesses for CVC. Most access to this vein is performed percutaneously with ultrasound guidance. Anatomical landmarks include Sedillot's triangle, which is bounded medially by the sternal head of the sternocleidomastoid muscle, laterally by the clavicular head of the sternocleidomastoid, and inferiorly by the superior border of the medial third of the clavicle (Fig. 8.1). The internal jugular vein is located at the apex of Sedillot's triangle and can be cannulated with a central, posterior, or anterior approach [9]. The internal jugular vein has anatomical variations that must be considered, given it is the most utilised site for CVC [10].

The subclavian vein is another option for CVC placement. Anatomically, it may represent one of the most challenging sites for cannulation due to the proximity of the lung and clavicle. However, some studies report better outcomes concerning infectious and thrombotic complications than other approaches (e.g. femoral vein) [11]. The typical location of the subclavian vein is the

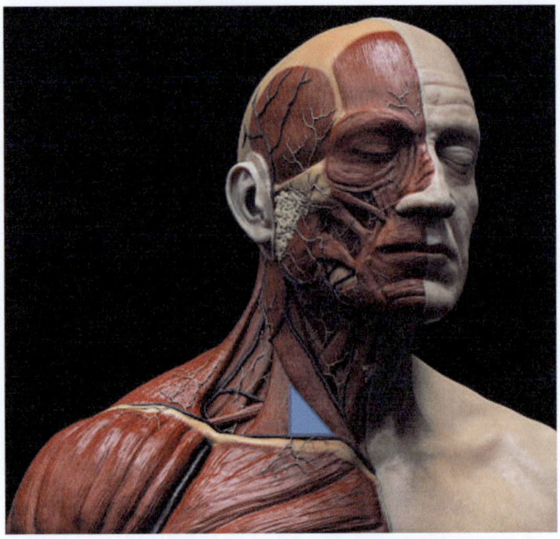

Fig. 8.1 Sedillot's triangle

medial third of the dorsal side of the clavicle. It lies superior to the first rib, inferior to the clavicle, and under the subclavius muscle. There are two approaches to the subclavian vein: infraclavicular and supraclavicular. The subclavian site is not the first choice for vein cannulation because bleeding complications are hard to assess and monitor, and local pressure is less effective.

The femoral vein is a common access point for CVC. Although frequently utilised, especially for radiological interventions, it may have a higher rate of complications when used for long-term catheterisation [12]. The femoral vein is usually cannulated just below the inguinal ligament. Its location is just medial to the femoral artery, which is generally easily located by palpation or ultrasound.

An alternative site for CVC insertion is the axillary vein. This can be an alternative to the internal jugular or subclavian veins and can be chosen when upper-body access is needed. Still, internal jugular and subclavian veins are not feasible. Anatomically, the axillary vein becomes the subclavian vein after passing the lateral border of the first rib. The axillary vein, usually located with ultrasound, allows more accessible access to the vena cava and right atrium with a lower potential for bleeding complications and brachial plexus injuries compared to more medial approaches [13].

ECG-guided positioning of CVC has been described. This technique aids physicians in determining the length of the catheter to be positioned. Besides empirical techniques, where the length is decided based on anatomical characteristics, ECG can be used because a CVC in an erroneous position may lead to arrhythmia, typically when entering the right atrium [14]. This technique may be beneficial in emergency settings, where saving time for X-ray confirmation is essential.

Placement of Intravenous Central Catheter in an Emergency Setting

Time-dependent decisions in an emergency setting limit the use of radiologic tools to locate a vein and perform uneventful VC positioning effectively. Furthermore, especially in cases of massive bleeding, central access may collapse, making VC positioning challenging. In these cases, a surgical approach to CVC placement might be helpful, safer, and faster if provided by skilled personnel.

In an emergency, a non-tunnelled catheter is typically chosen to provide life-saving fluids and drugs. These catheters, such as temporary non-tunnelled haemodialysis/pheresis catheters, multi-lumen catheters, and large-bore introducer sheaths, are not meant for chronic use and should be replaced within a few days of positioning.

Typical emergency settings include the following:

- Traumatic injuries
- Cannulation for extra corporeal membrane oxygenation
- Septic or haemodynamic shock
- Need for cardioactive, fast-acting drugs
- Need for rapid vital parameter monitoring
- Need for massive fluid administration or blood component transfusion
- Acute haemodialysis/plasmapheresis

In conclusion, the open-access approach to CVC is rare. Today, an ultrasound-guided approach is preferable and suggested by many international guidelines. An open approach should be cautiously chosen in adult patients and may be an option for rare emergency situations or repeated ultrasound-guided failure.

Intraosseous Access for Resuscitation and Emergency Situations

The need to obtain venous access is often a challenge for the clinician. Ultrasound has radically changed clinical approach strategies in standard conditions and emergency/urgent situations. However, there are some circumstances where ultrasound is not feasible, either due to unavailability, technical limitations, or the patient's clinical conditions that do not allow its use. In all these situations, the need to obtain valid, stable, efficient, and rapid access is met by the placement of intraosseous access. This method is not so modern but has been optimised in recent years. Initially developed for out-of-hospital and paediatric emergencies, it is now increasingly used and widespread in hospital settings and not just in emergency contexts. Many studies highlight the safety, efficacy, and simplicity of the intraosseous vascular approach to administering fluids and medications in numerous clinical situations [15–28].

The epiphyses of long bones consist of a thin layer of compact bone and abundant spongy tissue. Inside the medullary cavity of the proximal and distal epiphyses, there is an extensive system of rigid and non-collapsible vessels. These vessels form an integral part of the circulatory system; therefore, everything infused into the vessels of the diaphyseal cavity reaches the systemic circulation. No pharmacokinetic differences exist between intraosseous and direct intravascular administration [29]. Intraosseous administration reaches the right atrium with an average time of 2.42 s [30]. It is also important to note that the pressure within the medullary space can vary from 22% to 40% of systemic pressure [28, 31, 32] (Fig. 8.2).

Indications

The indications for placing intraosseous access are the same as those for identifying peripheral venous access. The fundamental considerations

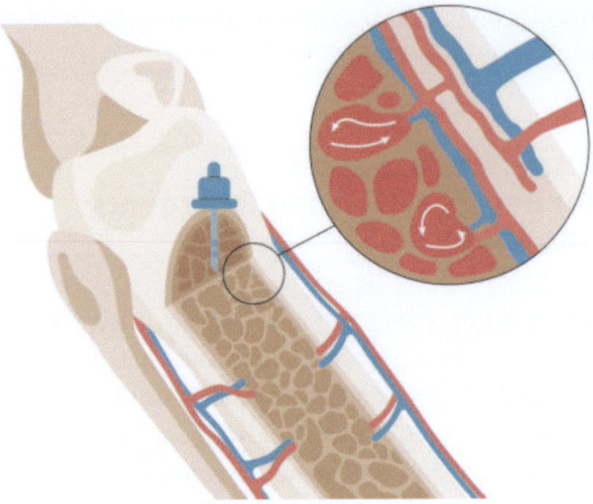

Fig. 8.2 Bone structure: vessels inside the medullary cavity

determining when an intraosseous device should be used include the urgent need for vascular access in acute conditions, chronic comorbidities, or anatomical difficulties (e.g. in paediatric patients) that complicate the placement of such peripheral or central intravenous access. Intraosseous access should not be placed solely for convenience when peripheral intravenous access can be easily obtained. However, the AHA and ERC guidelines on cardiopulmonary resuscitation indicate its use after two failed attempts to obtain peripheral access or as the first option in patients with complex or impossible access [33–35]. Considering that it is a simple, rapid technique whose success is independent of the patient's volemic status, the primary indication is the need to quickly infuse drugs and fluids in emergencies (cardiac arrest, shock) for adult and paediatric patients. However, intraosseous access represents an alternative for all patients with a problematic history of venous access due to comorbidities such as obesity, diabetes, chemotherapy, or drug abuse. It is essential to highlight that intraosseous devices allow for collecting bone marrow samples for laboratory analysis [36], blood sampling, and the infusion of radiological contrast fluids. Almost any drug can be administered, achieving the same pharmacokinetic performance and therapeutic effects as a peripheral intravenous infusion [37, 38].

Contraindications

Considering the limitations and conditions of use related to individual intraosseous devices, contraindications can be divided into absolute and relative. Among the *ABSOLUTE* contraindications, we find the following:

- Bone fractures, as they would cause direct extravasation of the administered drug or fluid; it is sufficient to select the insertion point on a non-fractured limb.
- Inability to correctly identify anatomical landmarks.
- Unsuccessful attempts to place intraosseous access within the previous 48 h at the same insertion site, as these would again cause direct extravasation.
- Orthopaedic prostheses implanted near the chosen insertion site; it is sufficient to select the insertion point in an anatomical area without a prosthesis.
- Skin infections near the chosen insertion site.
- Osteoporosis and osteomyelitis.

Among the *RELATIVE* contraindications to be evaluated based on clinical needs and situations:

- Severe obesity
- Burns of the skin area at the insertion site
- Previous placement of an intraosseous access at the same site
- Positive history of osteopenia and osteogenesis imperfecta, conditions that would increase the risk of iatrogenic fractures or drug extravasation [29]

Complications

Complications related to the placement of intraosseous access occur in less than 1% of cases [39, 40]. In the past, the main complication was osteomyelitis. Today, with the spread of the technique and the availability of modern devices, extravasation is the most frequent issue. If recognised immediately, it has insignificant consequences; however, if not promptly identified, it can lead to severe compartment syndromes.

In general, to reduce the risk of the described complications, it is advisable to undergo specific training on intraosseous access and never administer intraosseously at pressures exceeding 300 mmHg.

Therefore, the main complications are the following:

- *Compartment syndrome*: Caused by infusions into the soft tissues outside the vascular bed, leading to vascular and nerve damage that can result in tissue necrosis. To avoid it, it is essential to monitor the proper functioning of the infusion line, look for signs of extravasation, and stop the infusion immediately. To reduce its incidence, it is crucial to adhere to the correct placement technique and constantly monitor the effectiveness of the infusions.
- *Osteomyelitis*: Numerous studies have sought a correlation between intraosseous access and osteomyelitis. The reported incidence varies from 0% to 0.6%.
- *Embolism*: Thromboembolism is not a common complication (only one case described in the literature, with an uncertain correlation). The same applies to gas embolism; sporadic and uncertain cases have been described. However, avoiding air entry through the intraosseous needle is a good practice, and it should be capped when not in use. Fat embolism is related to the initial flush and infusion pressures; the effects of this event, however, are clinically insignificant [41].
- *Effects on bone and its growth*: No evidence exists of the toxicity of drugs administered intraosseously and their potential effects on bone marrow quality. In the paediatric population, it is advisable to avoid damaging growth plates. A fibrin plug seals the bone punctured by the intraosseous access placement within 48 h. Complete bone repair, however, can take weeks to months [42, 43].

Fluids and Medications

The intraosseous space represents vascular access in every respect. Therefore, through intraosseous access, fluids of any type (crystalloids, colloids, blood products, and hypertonic solutions) can be infused. The infusion rate varies depending on the patient's characteristics, the access site used, and the type of needle.

Medications can be administered intraosseously at the exact dosages and concentrations as intravenous administrations (Table 8.1) [29, 34, 44, 45]. Regarding chemotherapeutic agents, there is no clear recommendation for their administration, although cases have been described. In these instances, particular care is recommended, along with a saline flush, to remove any drug residues from the medullary space.

Landmarks

Five possible insertion sites for intraosseous needle placement (Fig. 8.3) were chosen based on patient characteristics and available devices.

1. *Proximal tibia* (Fig. 8.4)

For a prone patient, slightly flex the knee and locate the tibial tuberosity. Move 2-3 cm downwards (1 cm in paediatric patients) and 1 cm medially. It can accept up to 1 L/h [48]. In adults, insert the needle perpendicularly to the bone surface. In paediatric patients, angle the needle caudally by 10°–15° to reduce the risk of growth plate injury.

2. *Distal tibia* (Fig. 8.5)

Identify the medial malleolus and move 3 cm upwards (1–2 cm in neonates/paediatric patients). In adults, insert the needle perpendicularly to the bone surface. In paediatric patients, angle the needle cranially by 10°–15° to reduce the risk of growth plate injury.

3. *Humeral* (Fig. 8.6)

With the arm adducted, locate the surgical neck of the humerus and identify the humeral head. Insert the needle at a 45° angle to the horizontal plane. The needle can accept up to 5 L/h [48].

Table 8.1 Medications that can be administered intraosseously (with evident references from the literature)

Adenosine	Dexamethasone	Fosphenytoin	Phenytoin
Adrenaline	Dextrose (10%to 50%)	Furosemide	Pneumococcal vaccine
Albumin	Diazoxide	Gentamicin	Potassium chloride
Alfentanil	Digoxin	Isoprenaline	Promethazine
Alteplase	Diltiazem	Ketamine	Propofol
Aminophylline	Diphenhydramine	Labetalol	Recombinant factor VII
Amiodarone	Dobutamine	Levitiracetam	Remifentanil
Ampicillin	Dopamine	Meningococcal vaccine	Rocuronium
Anti-tetanus (serum)	Ephedrine	Lidocaine	Sodium bicarbonate
Atracurium	Etomidate	Linezolid	Succinylcholine
Atropine	Fentanyl	Lorazepam	Sufentanil
Aztreonam	Floxacillin	Magnesium sulphate	Tenecteplase
Benzylpenicillin (PenicillinG)	Fluconazole	Mannitol	Tetanus immunoglobulin
Bretylium	Flumazenil	Methylprednisolone	Thiamine
Calcium (chloride and gluconate)	Haloperidol	Mdazolam	Thiopental
Cefazolin	Heparin	Mivacurium	Tobramycin
Cefotaxime	Hydroxocobalamin	Morpnine	Vancomycin
Ceftriaxone	Hydrocortisone	Naloxone	Vasopressin
Cisatracurium	Hydromorphone	Phenytoin	Vecuronium
Contrast media	Insulin	Phenobarbital	Vitamin K
Diazepam	Isoproterenol	Phenylephrine	Tranexamic acid

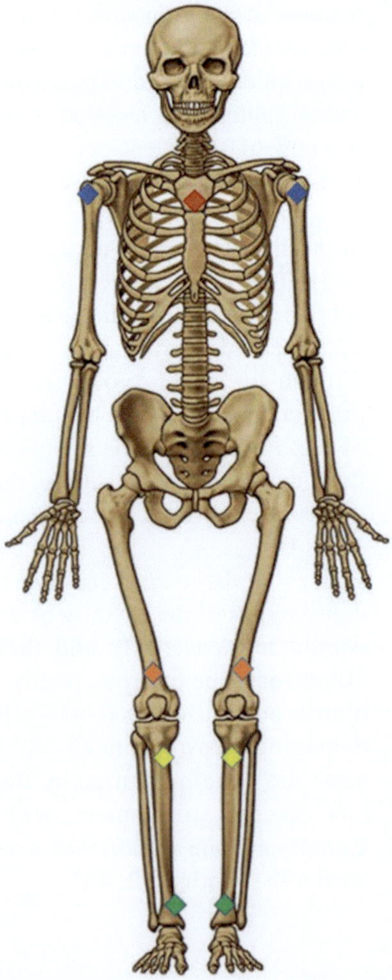

Fig. 8.3 Insertion sites for intraosseous needle. (Reproduced with permission from Bartl and Bartl [46])

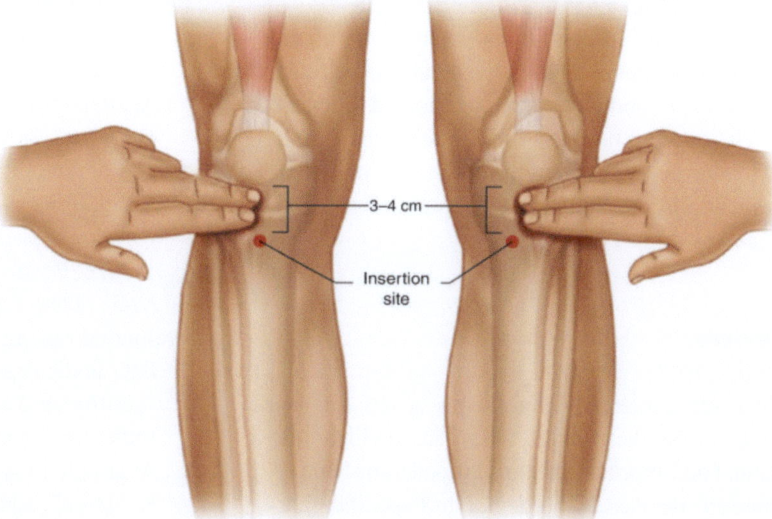

Fig. 8.4 Proximal tibia. (Reproduced with permission from Quibell and Yip [47])

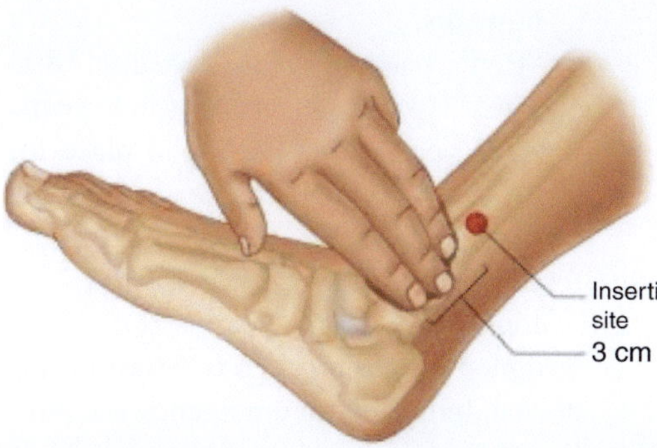

Fig. 8.5 Distal tibia. (Reproduced with permission from Quibell and Yip [47])

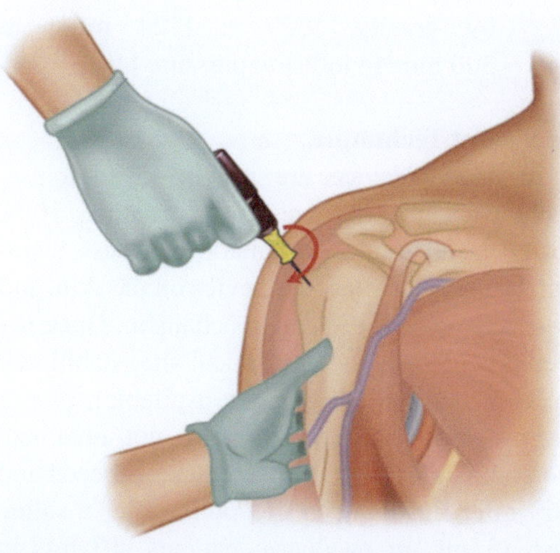

Fig. 8.6 Humeral landmark. (Reproduced with permission from Quibell and Yip [47])

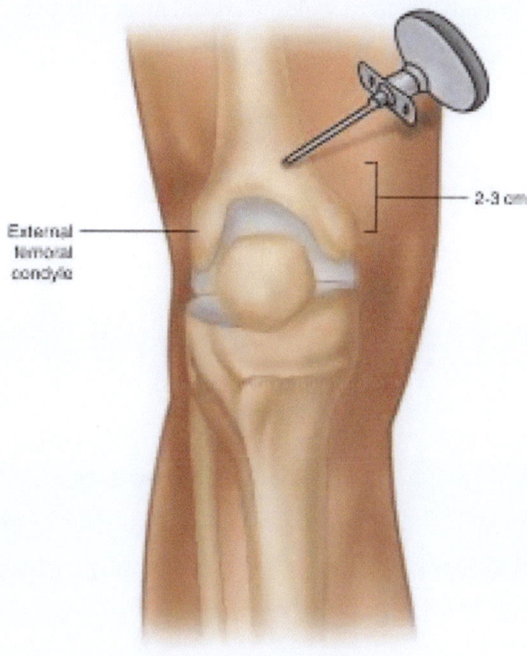

Fig. 8.7 Distal femur. (Reproduced with permission from Quibell and Yip [47])

4. *Distal femur* (Fig. 8.7)

Recommended in paediatric patients under 6 years old. Locate the patella. Move approximately 1 cm above the patella and 1–2 cm medial to the centre of the femur. Insert the needle at a 90° angle to the bone surface.

5. *Sternal* (Fig. 8.8)

Indicated only in conditions where none of the previous sites are usable (typically in military contexts) and only with dedicated devices. The optimal target is the centre of the sternal manubrium, between the interclavicular ligament and the insertion of the second rib. Can accept up to 10 L/h.

Devices

There are numerous intraosseous access devices available on the market. They are divided into manual and mechanical (spring-loaded or battery-powered) devices. Each device has specific characteristics that limit its use to certain landmarks. We will focus on mechanical devices, which are currently the most widespread and most effective.

1. *Spring-Loaded*
   (a) *BIG® (Persys Medical)*

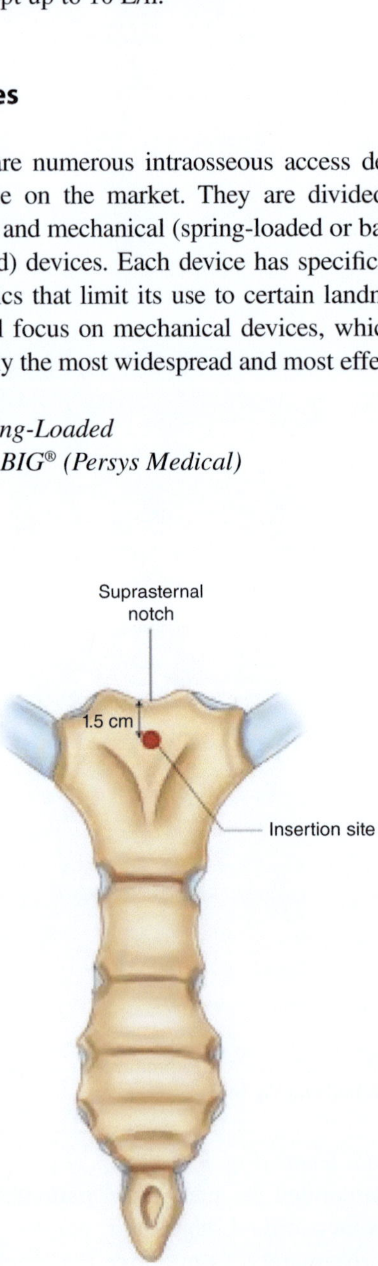

Fig. 8.8 Sternal landmark. (Reproduced with permission from Quibell and Yip [47])

Preloaded spring device. For adult and paediatric use. Indicated for emergency use only. It can remain in place for up to 24 h. Available in two versions:

- "Blue", adult (>12 years); 15 G size. Positionable in proximal tibia and humerus
- "Red", paediatric (0–12 years); 18 G size. Positionable in proximal tibia

(b) *NIO® (Persys Medical)*

Preloaded spring device. The evolution of BIG is distinguished by improved needle stability and adjustable insertion depth. Indicated for emergency use only. Available in two versions:

- "Blue", adult (>12 years); 15 G size. It can remain in place for up to 72 h. Positionable in proximal tibia and humerus.
- "Red", paediatric (3–12 years); 18 G size. Two depth steps (3–9 years; 9–12 years). Can remain in place for up to 24 h. Positionable in proximal tibia.

(c) *FAST1® and FASTR® (Pyng-Teleflex)*

For adult use (>12 years). Originally designed for military needs. Multi-needle device. Indicated for emergency use only. It can remain in place for up to 24 h. Available in two sizes (16 G and 18 G—only for FAST1). Positionable only in the sternal site. Infusion rate 1130 ± 692 mL/h by gravity, 5327 ± 1724 mL/h at 300 mmHg infusion pressure [49].

Placement Technique

Spring-loaded devices are straightforward to use. Their placement requires no more than 10 s. Locate the anatomical landmark for access, disinfect the skin site, place the device on the skin, and press to release the spring mechanism. Once the needle penetrates the anatomical site, stabilize it (specific fixation systems are available), blood/marrow aspiration (occasionally not obtained, even with correct needle placement; proceed and retry after flushing); at this point, after a saline flush (5 mL in paediatric patients, 10 mL in adults—to break bone trabeculae allowing diffusion of administered/infused substances), fluids can be infused (preferably using pressure bags) and medications administered (always followed by a saline flush).

2. *Battery-Powered*
   (a) *EZ-IO® (Teleflex)*
   Highly versatile, rapid, and precise tool. Currently, it is the only battery-powered intraosseous device. Consists of a multi-use drill (up to 500 insertions) with disposable needles. Indicated for emergency, urgent, or specific clinical needs. It can remain in place for up to 72 h (in Europe). Needles available in three different lengths (all 15 G):
   - 15 mm: For patients weighing 3–39 kg. Primarily for paediatric patients
   - 25 mm: For patients >3 kg. Primarily for tibial access in normal-sized patients
   - 45 mm: For patients >39 kg. Primarily for humeral access and tibial access in patients with high adipose tissue

   The humeral site is suitable for adult and paediatric patients. The proximal and distal tibial sites suit adult, paediatric, and neonatal patients. The distal femoral site is suitable for paediatric and neonatal patients (up to approximately 6 years old).
   (b) *EZ-IO® T.A.L.O.N. (Teleflex)*
   An EZ-IO version that also allows sternal placement, with a specific kit featuring a locator for anatomical landmarks. Infusion rate 9587 ± 2706 mL/h at 300 mmHg infusion pressure [50].

Placement Technique
EZ-IO is very simple to use and currently represents one of the best available options regarding effectiveness, safety, and convenience. Placement takes a maximum of 10 s. Select the anatomical landmark for access. Choose the most suitable needle (in addition to the abovementioned indications, ensure the first black notch on the needle is visible once the drill is aimed at the landmark point). Disinfect the skin site. Activate the drill until resistance is felt. Remove the drill and unscrew the introducer while firmly holding the needle. Connect the dedicated extension set, aspirate blood/marrow (occasionally not obtained, even with correct needle placement; therefore, retry after flushing), and subsequently inject a saline flush (10 mL for adults, 5 mL for children, ensuring the access capacity and absence of subcutaneous leakage). Stabilise the needle (the needle package includes a specific adhesive stabiliser).

REMEMBER!
- Always remember to evaluate the correct infusion and pay attention to any extravasations, which could cause compartment syndromes.
- NO flush = NO flow ➔ Always remember to flush the needle after positioning.
- Generally, the placement of an intraosseous needle is not painful and is comparable to the sensation experienced with a normal peripheral access. However, what can cause intense pain in conscious patients is the rapid injection of the saline flush. In these cases, if possible, slow administration of lidocaine is recommended (20–40 mg for adults; 0.5 mg/kg for paediatric patients) prior to the flush.

Infusion of fluids at normal pressures, on the other hand, does not cause pain or significant discomfort [51, 52].

Haemodialysis Access and Other Vascular Access Options

Introduction

A stable and sufficiently high blood flow in the extracorporeal system is essential for effective renal replacement therapy. In addition to other factors, this is determined by well-functioning vascular access. The dialysis catheters can be either *non-tunnelled* or *subcutaneously tunnelled* for long-term use. Large lumen non-tunnelled dialysis catheters are the primary access for acute kidney injury (AKI) patients in intensive care. Catheter design and material also affect the flow characteristics, such as insertion site and volume status. Short-term catheters should be used for acute haemodialysis and *for a limited time* in hospitalised patients. It should be planned to remove or convert each short-term catheter to a long-term one within a week. The use of temporary (non-tunnelled and non-cuffed) CVCs for haemodialysis should be limited to a maximum of 2 weeks because of the increased risk of infection, and their use should be considered only in patients with a need for urgent vascular access (in intensive care or case of urgent admission in the nephrology department) [53, 54].

Short-Term Central Venous Dialysis Catheters

The inner diameter of the catheter is a significant determinant of blood flow. The highly different lumen shapes among different catheters make comparisons on the inner diameter difficult, so only the outer diameter is given to clinicians. The maximum diameter has not yet been established; however, when the catheter is too large for the vein, it becomes an obstacle to flow and increases the risk of thrombosis and vessel wall trauma leading to an inflammatory reaction resulting in stenosis (Fig. 8.9). A 12–16 Fr catheter (1 French = 1/3 mm) is adequate for all dialysis modalities in the ICU. The material is polyurethane or silicone. The thin wall of the polyurethane catheter allows a larger inner diameter. The stiffness facilitates insertion but exposes to the theoretical risk of vascular or atrial trauma. All venous catheters, however, are thermoplastic and therefore become more flexible at body temperature and assume the vessel's shape. Silicone ones are flexible but difficult to insert. They traumatise the vessel less. The wall thickness is greater, and thus, the inner diameter is reduced. However, the material has little influence on the durability of a catheter, which usually should not exceed 2–3 weeks.

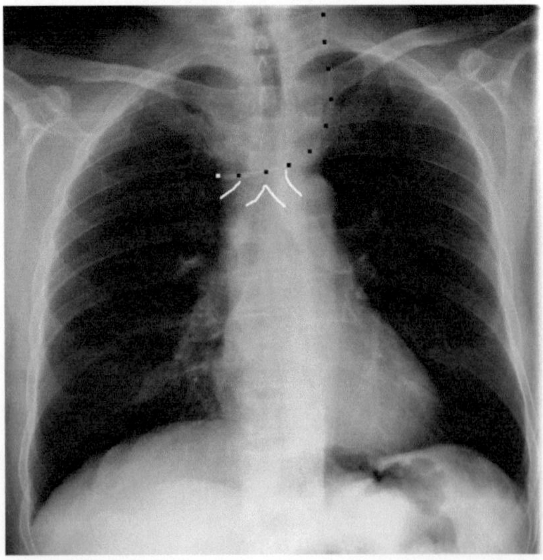

Fig. 8.9 Short-term dialysis CVC (16 cm) inserted in left internal jugular vein with malposition due to its too short length. The angle of incidence with the vein wall is >40°

"Basic Principles

Dialysis catheters usually have at least two lumens with two colour-coded red and blue ports (Fig. 8.10). By convention, the red port identifies the arterial lumen draining blood from the body (proximal/lateral opening) and the blue port identifies the venous lumen for blood reinfusion back to the patient from the dialysis machine (distal opening). Sometimes, the flow can be reversed if it is limited in conventional directions. Non-tunnelled three-lumen short-term dialysis catheters are also available, which reduces the need for additional central catheters and peripheral accesses. The third port is between the blue and red ports and is usually used for blood sampling and administering fluids or drugs.

Puncture Sites

Regarding vessel topography, the *right internal jugular vein* is the most favourable puncture site, as a central position of the catheter tip is possible via a relatively short and straight route. Catheter placement via the subclavian vein is associated with many complications and should be avoided wherever possible. In case internal jugular veins are unavailable for cannulation, axillary ultrasound-guided access should be preferred over subclavian access. This prevents catheter compression between the first rib and the clavicle, which can lead to malfunction or fracture of the catheter. This event is typical of subclavian

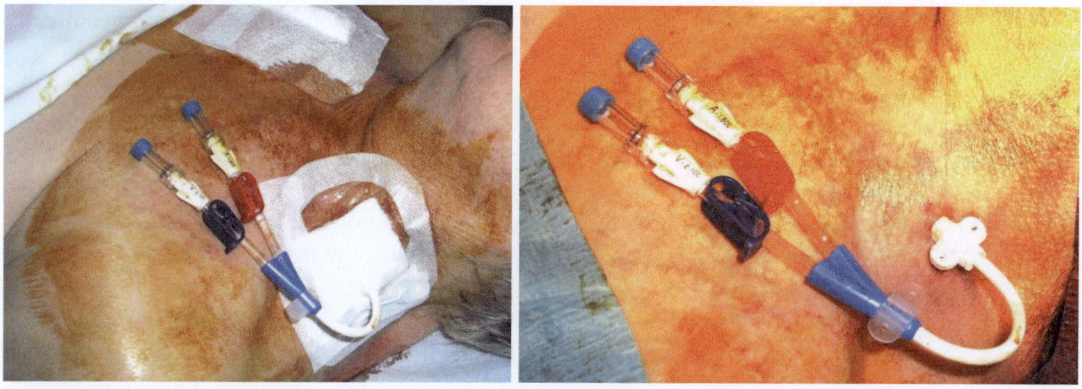

Fig. 8.10 Short-term pre-curved dialysis catheter (Teleflex 12F pre-curved 20 cm). Increased patient comfort. In post-procedural radiological control, it can be confused with a tunnelled long-term catheter

vein catheterisations (pinch-off sign) [55]. In the ultrasound-guided infraclavicular approach to the *axillary vein*, the catheter is inserted into the vein well before the clavicle-costal passage, making it difficult for pinch-off. *Femoral* catheters without a cuff should preferably be used in intensive care or bedridden patients. Regarding hygiene, catheterisation of the femoral vein is the most unsuitable option. Therefore, prolonged catheter positioning times should be avoided. Femoral catheters should be of sufficient length to have high flows and to minimise recirculation. A catheter that does not reach the inferior vena cava often does not reach 300 mL/min. With longer catheters (30–35 cm), the target position is more easily reached, although there is more resistance due to the length of the catheter [56]. Contraindications to CVC in the femoral vein include pathologies of the femoral or iliac vessels or previous surgery/reconstruction, hygienic reasons (e.g. unresolved chronic diarrhoea), and morbid obesity (BMI > 35 kg/m^2).

Flow Problems

Depending on the catheter position, insufficient volume status can lead to suction problems, which can repeatedly lead to interruptions in therapy and, therefore, negatively impact the procedure's effectiveness and the filter operating life. Reversing the connections on the catheter is not always an effective solution. Depending on the catheter design and position, this can lead to a backflow of just-purified blood into the dialyser (recirculation), significantly minimising dialysis effectiveness. A cautious reduction in blood flow velocity or fluid withdrawal is better, although not without disadvantages. For femoral catheters, poor flows are usually observed when the patient is in a sitting position.

Factors Determining the Choice of Insertion Site for the Temporary, Non-tunnelled Haemodialysis Catheter

- For right internal jugular vein or anonymous right vein: patients recovering from recent major abdominal surgery, e.g. aortic aneurysm; active infections in the groin area; acute diarrhoea or fungal infections; previous vascular surgery (e.g. bypass) involving the groin or lower extremity; morbid obesity. Jugular/anonym access should be considered for patients with BMI > 28 to avoid maceration and colonisation at the femoral vascular access site.
- For the common femoral vein: chronic dialysis patients with a fistula or graft are present or likely shortly. In the presence of an inexperienced operator or when an ultrasound device is unavailable, the patient requires emergent dialysis. Lastly, severe coagulopathy is an indication of femoral vein cannulation. For patients with BMI < 28, the most recent studies found no difference in the incidence of infection compared with the supraclavicular site. In contrast, in patients with BMI < 24, the

Table 8.2 Regarding site choice, we can summarise as follows: first choice is for the right supraclavicular site, second for the femoral vein, third for the left supraclavicular site, and last choice for the axillary vein, preferring the dominant side

Preferred insertion site of short-term CICC for acute haemodialysis and required length	Catheter length
Right supraclavicular approach	15 cm
Left supraclavicular approach	25 cm
Right or left femoral vein	25–30 cm
Right axillary vein	20–25 cm
Left axillary vein	25–30 cm

dressing will be challenging to adhere due to bony prominences.

- For left internal jugular or left anonymous vein: contraindications to dx internal jugular or dx anonymous vein and femoral veins.
- For axillary/subclavian veins: contraindications to the internal jugular and femoral veins. Prefer axillary veins over subclavian veins (Table 8.2).

Procedure of Short-Term Dialysis Catheter Placement

- Thus, the preferred puncture site is the ultrasound-guided access to the anonymous vein or the right internal jugular vein posterior to the lateral head of the sternocleidomastoid muscle, 1–2 cm above the clavicle (Jernigan-Pittiruti route). The introducer needle is visualised in the plane, and the jugular/animal vein is visualised in the short axis. Before venipuncture, the patency and compressibility of the vessel are assessed sonographically to rule out stenosis and thrombosis, especially in the case of previous central cannulation.
- The metal guide is inserted through the 18 G introducer needle. Ultrasound verifies the correct direction of the guide wire and can confirm the venous placement of the wire before dilation [5].
- In dialysis catheterisation (large calibre), performing a skin incision a few millimetres immediately lateral to the metal guide is essential. The tissue dilator is introduced until a loss of resistance is detected.
- The central venous catheter is inserted directly over the metal guidewire.
- The catheter tip position is checked immediately with intracavitary electrocardiography or transthoracic ultrasound with contrast medium (bubble test). Fluoroscopy may be used in dubious cases. With pulmonary ultrasonography, the ipsilateral lung is checked. In doubtful cases, lung verification should be performed several hours later to exclude a pneumothorax. A post-procedural radiological verification does not allow immediate correction of any malpositioning.
- In the case of dialysis catheters, flow from each lumen should be verified by aspiration test and subsequent flushing. Before device stabilisation is performed, the anticoagulant solution is injected at the specified volume on each catheter lumen.

Tip Location

For haemodialysis CICC, the correct position of the CICC-tip is at the mid-right atrium to avoid vessel and right atrial trauma or complications [57].

For lower body insertion sites, the correct position of the FICC-tip is at the inferior vena cava above the diaphragm level [57].

Methods for confirming the position of the catheter tip include chest radiography, fluoroscopy, or continuous electrocardiography [5].

Post-procedural Controls

Post-insertion imaging should be considered to avoid malpositioning of CVCs [56]. The correct position of the CVC should be in the centre of the right atrium to avoid vascular and atrial trauma and subsequent complications. To avoid the costs and risks of fluoroscopy, it is now recommended that an effective and accurate *intra-procedural methodology* such as the intracavitary ECG technique be used for haemodialysis catheters, followed by radiological monitoring only in unclear clinical situations.

Short-Term Dialysis Catheter Removal

In dialysis catheter removal, gas embolism should be prevented in practice by performing finger pressure on the venipuncture site until haemostasis is achieved; then, a sterile occlusive dressing should be applied over the catheter exit site. The occlusive dressing should remain in place for 72 h to prevent delayed gas embolism. The dressing should be checked regularly to ensure it remains intact and leak-free during this time. The best system currently available to reduce the risk of gas embolism is the application of cyanoacrylate glue immediately after removing the central venous catheter.

Hygiene and Dressing Changes

Concerning catheter placement and the requirements for dressing changes and handling, the same hygiene recommendations should be followed as for central venous catheters. However, if discontinuous renal replacement procedures are used, the dressing should be changed after each dialysis. However, given the large catheter lumen and the cannulated large vessels, securing the catheter is essential to prevent accidental removal. In general, the catheter manipulation rate should be kept as low as possible, which is why these accesses should ideally not be used for infusions and blood sampling, even during the dialysis-free interval. If catheter-associated infection with septicemia is suspected, the infected catheter should be removed, the tip examined microbiologically if possible and reinserted elsewhere (Table 8.3).

Long-Term Central Venous Dialysis Catheters (Tunnelled Dialysis Catheters)

If dialysis is expected to be required for a more extended period, the use of a tunnelled dialysis catheter can be considered, as the infection rates are significantly lower [59]. However, it is only recommended if the patient has a stable infection, as changing the catheter is much more complicated.

Numerous catheters of different designs and materials are available on the market. The catheter is inserted using percutaneous intervention using the Seldinger technique. The preferred vessel here is also the right internal or external jugular vein. The tip of the catheter is placed in the right atrium, whereby the tunnelled course

Table 8.3 Summary of characteristics of short-term dialysis central venous catheter

Venous access of choice	*Right anonymous vein* or the *right internal jugular vein*. The subclavian vein and the axillary vein should not be used for dialysis/apheresis, both because of their small calibre compared to the anonymous and internal jugular veins (risk of venous thrombosis) and because a possible thrombosis or stenosis of the subclavian-axillary axis could impair the creation of an AV fistula on that side. *Femoral access* in dialysis catheterisation (FICC) is the second choice after right supraclavicular access (anonymous vein or internal jugular vein). The right femoral vein is preferred as a first choice because it is shorter and less tortuous
Tip location	The distal end of the CICC should ideally be positioned in the right atrium, 1–2 cm below the junction between the superior vena cava and the right atrium. The catheter should be advanced in the femoral vein (FICC) beyond the bifurcation of the common iliac vein until it reaches the inferior vena cava. A catheter that does not reach the inferior vena cava often does not achieve a flow of 300 mL/min
Duration	A non-tunnelled dialysis catheter should be removed as soon as possible and replaced with a long-lasting tunnelled catheter. Because of the risk of infection, use should be limited to a maximum of 2 weeks (KDOQI 2019). Consider their use only in patients with need for emergent access (INS 2024)
Management	Patency maintained with *anticoagulant lock*. After each access or weekly. The volume in millilitres is printed on the lumen of the catheter. The catheter hub should be cleaned (when connecting and disconnecting the catheter) with a chlorhexidine-based solution. If chlorhexidine is contraindicated (e.g. sensitivity and allergy), povidone-iodine solution (preferably with alcohol) is a reasonable substitute and should be used [58]

between the exit site from the vessel and the exit from the skin creates a distance that protects against bacterial contamination.

Puncture Sites

If possible, long-term dialysis catheters should not be placed on the same side of a maturing fistula. Special care should be taken in avoiding femoral catheters in patients who are candidates or candidates for renal transplantation. The preferred insertion site of a cuffed haemodialysis venous catheter is still the *right internal jugular vein*. Patients requiring *femoral* access usually have limited mobility, so tunnelling does not significantly restrict their daily life. The tunnel can be placed downward on the anterior surface of the thigh or upward on the abdomen if downward tunnelling excessively limiting movement. With subcutaneous tunnelling on the abdomen, attention must be paid to the belt line, which may be uncomfortable for the patient and may cause kinking of the catheter. Without contraindications, prior pathology (e.g. central stenosis) or intervention (e.g. pacemaker), CVC insertion on the right side is preferable to the left side due to more direct anatomy. If one side has pathology that limits AV access creation but allows for CVC insertion, this side should be used for the CVC to preserve the other side for AV access creation. If the internal jugular veins are not previous or of sufficient size, it is better to puncture the *axillary vein* at the level of the infraclavicular fossa. The subclavian vein should be avoided as it runs under a bony structure (clavicle), is not ultrasound visible, and is compressible in case of bleeding (Fig. 8.11).

Choice of Material

Using pre-bent catheters with anterograde tunnelling in jugular venous accesses reduces the risk of neck kinking. In the case of femoral or axillary venous accesses, it is preferable to use straight catheters. It is necessary to have different lengths available to reach the right atrium with the tip in all sizes of patients. In small patients, less than 15 cm is often required to get

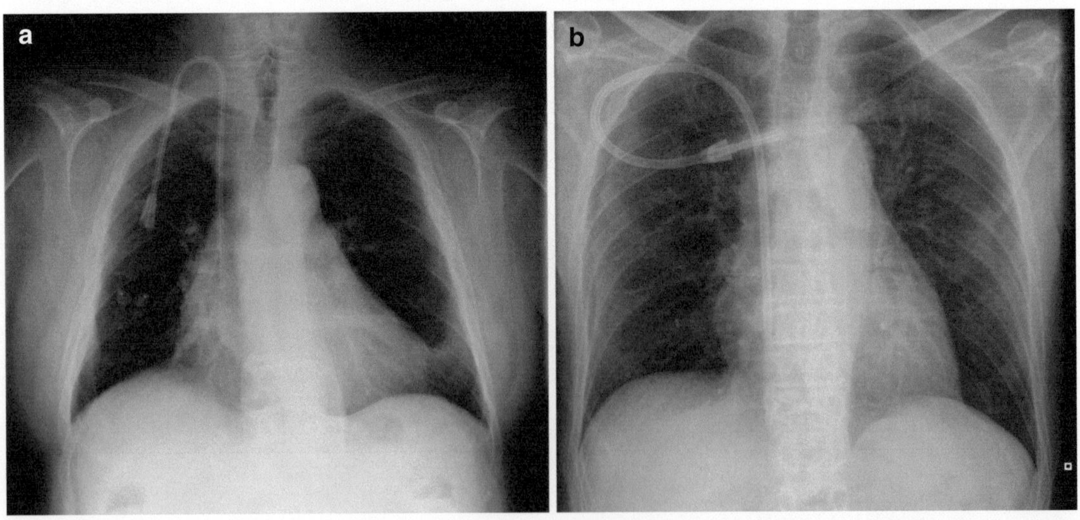

Fig. 8.11 (**a**) Anterograde pre-curved tunnelled dialysis catheter (Bard HemoStar® 14.5F 24 cm) inserted in the right internal jugular vein and tunnelled on the chest. Tip in the right atrium. Well-functioning. (**b**) Straight anterograde cuffed tunnelled dialysis catheter (BARD HemoStar® 14.5F 28 cm) inserted in the right axillary vein and tunnelled towards the middle of the thorax. Tip in the right atrium. Well-functioning. (Department of Anaesthesiology, Bolzano Hospital)

the right atrium with the right jugular access. For femoral accesses, special straight catheters with a length of up to 75 cm (cuff tip 55 cm) are needed to tunnel and correctly reach the right atrium. For catheters with retrograde tunnelling, it is likewise essential to have different lengths available. Catheters that are too long would result in long tunnels that predispose to malpositioning and often do not achieve an optimal skin exit site. Currently, no advantage of one type of catheter over another has been demonstrated in the long term, although many studies are underway in this area. Catheters allowing high flows (350 mL/min with pre-pump pressures no more negative than 250 mmHg) are preferred. The choice of catheter should be based on local experience, objectives in use, and costs (Figs. 8.12 and 8.13).

Anterograde Tunnelling

In this case, tunnelling is performed after positioning and ultrasound verification of the position of the metal guide in the selected vein. Anterograde tunnelling is performed from the skin exit point on the thoracic wall/thigh and is directed to the level of the lowest portion of the space (10–15 mm) created at the neck/inguinal level around the venipuncture site (around the metal guide). The neck/inguinal opening in anterograde tunnels must be sufficiently large to simultaneously contain both the catheter and the peel-away introducer-dilator.

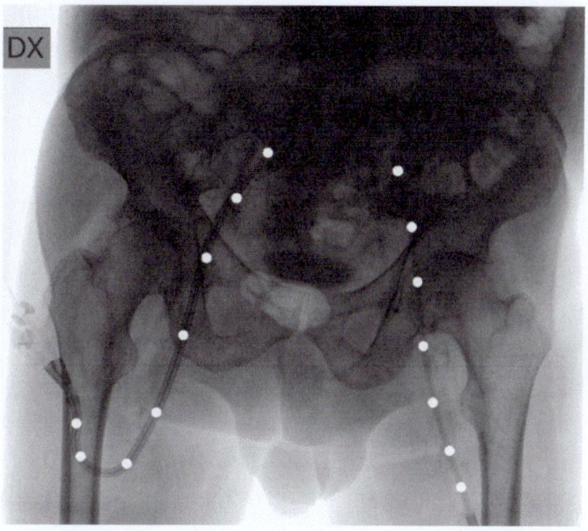

Fig. 8.12 Tunnelled dialysis catheter in the right femoral vein. Short-term dialysis catheter in the left femoral vein. Both malfunctioned as they were too short, with tips in the respective iliac veins

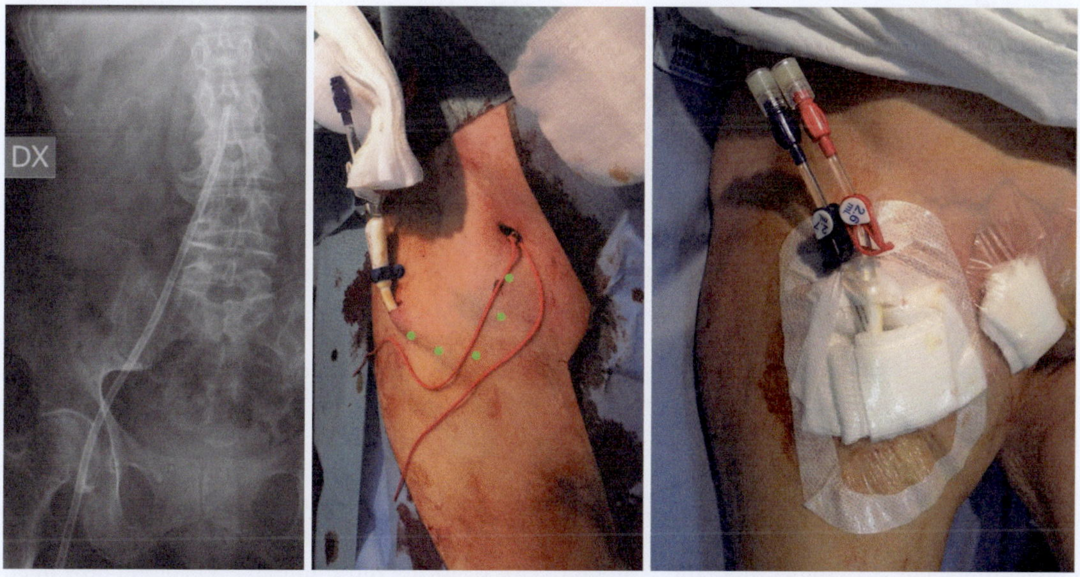

Fig. 8.13 An anterograde tunnelled dialysis catheter (Angiodynamics 14.5F 40 cm) was inserted in the right femoral vein and tunnelled laterally on the thigh. Tip in inferior vena cava. Well-functioning

Retrograde Tunnelling

In this case, the peel-away introducer-dilator is inserted immediately after venous puncture and insertion and ultrasound verification of the metal guide. The surgical incision around the guide must be sufficiently large to contain the peel-away. After inserting the catheter into the vein, the tunnel is created from the entry point into the vein in the direction of the cutaneous exit point, which can be on the chest wall or on the thigh.

Anterograde-Retrograde Insertion Over the Wire

In this case, the peel-away introducer-dilator is not used, but the catheter is inserted directly over the metal guidewire after dilatation with tissue dilatators. Tunnelling can be either anterograde or retrograde. The surgical dissection is less extensive, and the risk of gas embolism is lower (this is why many peel-away dilatators are provided with a valve). Usually, the silicone catheter is made more rigid by the presence of stylets in the lumens of the catheter within which the metal guide runs. After verification of the position of the tip, the metal guide wire is removed and subsequently, the stylets.

Tip Position

The tip of the CVC should be placed in the middle and deep right atrium. In this position, CVC dysfunction and infection were similar for left versus right approaches. KDOQI considers it reasonable that if fluoroscopy is not used to insert a tunnelled CVC, alternative imaging ensures the CVC tip has been correctly placed [58].

Management of the Tunnelled Dialysis Catheter

It is reasonable to clean the catheter hub when connecting and disconnecting the catheter with a chlorhexidine solution. If chlorhexidine is contraindicated (e.g. due to hypersensitivity or allergy), an iodine-povidone solution (preferably with alcohol) should be used. The dressing should also be changed after each dialysis, with a thorough inspection of the exit site to detect infection. When changing the catheter dressing, the skin surrounding the catheter exit site should be cleaned with a chlorhexidine-based solution (alternatively iodo-povidone with alcohol). Radiological diagnostics should be considered in case of catheter malfunction that does not respond to conservative procedures and administration of tissue plasminogen activator (TPA) [58]. Antimicrobial ointments may be used on the exit site [57, 60].

Intraluminal Agents to Prevent Central Venous Dialysis Catheter Malfunction (Short- and Long-Term with Cuff)

Dialysis catheters should be flushed with 0.9% 20 mL physiological saline using the pressure/pause technique on the syringe and filled with a particular lock solution ("catheter lock") following internal hospital standards. Filling volumes are always indicated on the catheter by the manufacturer. This procedure must be performed after dialysis and each use of the catheter. The anticoagulant solution must be removed from the catheter before its use and before its removal. Accidental injection of a "citrate block" must be avoided by sufficient aspiration or volume-accurate instillation, as this can induce significant cardiac arrhythmia depending on the concentration! Haemodialysis CVCs can be located with low concentration (<5%) of heparin or citrate solution. However, heparin and citrate are the most widely used, as they are believed to have an antimicrobial and antithrombotic effect. Locking of CVCs with tissue plasminogen activator (tPA) for prophylactic reasons once a week should be considered to reduce the risk of catheter occlusion [57]. KDOQI recommends using alteplase (2 mg) or urokinase plus citrates 4% per limb for restoring intraluminal CVC blood flow in an occluded CVC [58].

Catheter-Related Bloodstream Infection (CRBSI) Definition

Clinical manifestations and at least one positive blood culture result from a peripheral source (*dialysis circuit* or *vein*) and no other apparent source, with either positive semiquantitative (>15 CFU/catheter segment, hub or tip) or quantitative (>10^2 CFU/catheter segment, e.g. hub or tip) culture, whereby the same organism (species and antibiogram) is isolated from the catheter segment (e.g. hub or tip) and a peripheral source (dialysis circuit or vein) blood sample. If available, the following would be supportive: simultaneous quantitative cultures of blood samples with a ratio of ≥3:1 (catheter hub/tip vs peripheral [dialysis circuit/vein]) and differential period of catheter culture versus peripheral blood culture positivity of 2 h. The management of an infected catheter depends on the patient's health, dialysis, and vascular access and should follow the detailed guidelines. Options include CVC exchange by guidewire, CVC removal and reinsertion, CVC salvage, and concurrent antibiotic lock (particularly if the CVC is considered to be the patient's final access) [58].

CVC Dysfunction

Persistent CVC dysfunction may be due to intraluminal or pericatheter thrombus or development of a fibrin sheath. Fibrin sheaths may develop during CVC insertion, recruiting platelets and other coagulation factors and promoting leukocyte adherence. Over days to months, collagen is deposited near the tip of the venous vessel wall where the CVC is located. If clotting exceeds the endogenous fibrinolytic system's capacity, subsequent CVC thrombosis will ensue. The main types of CVC-related thrombi include intraluminal thrombus, CVC tip thrombus, and fibrin sheath thrombus, the most common type. Management is directed at these types of thrombi.

Treatment of CVC Dysfunction

The treatments can be categorised by the type of intervention: bedside manoeuvres and medical and mechanical interventions. Medical interventions are further subdivided into conservative manoeuvres and pharmacologic interventions per se. Mechanical interventions are also subdivided into fibrin sheath disruption, catheter exchange, and CVC removal with replacement.

1. Bedside manoeuvres

Patient repositioned lateral or Trendelenburg position, rapid saline flushes, and lumen reversal.

2. Pharmacologic interventions (conservative management)

Thrombolytic agents: TPA 1 mg/mL or Urokinase 5000 IU/mL (dwell over 40 min). Treatment success is not significantly different between the two thrombolytic agents.

3. Mechanical interventions

Catheter exchange (kinking, tip malposition, occlusion). Older CVCs will likely have fibrous tissue formed around the cuff, necessitating subcutaneous dissection and subsequent replacement with a new tunnelled CVC. It is necessary to obliterate the fibrin sheath before performing the CVC exchange to prevent early failure of the CVC after exchange. This is useful and important, especially for patients with limited central venous access sites.

Fibrin sheath stripping with a loop snare. The most common treatment for malfunctioning tunnelled haemodialysis catheters is fibrin stripping. For fibrin stripping, a guide wire is advanced through the distal lumen of the tunnelled dialysis catheter. Through femoral venous access, an introducer sheath is placed, and a snare loop is advanced into the inferior vena cava, over the guide wire and then over the catheter. The snare loop is tightened around the tunnelled catheter and drawn down to scrape any thrombus or fibrin sheaths off the catheter. This process is repeated until pulling the loop snare over the catheter becomes easier, indicating that most of the debris has been removed [61] (Fig. 8.14).

Internal snare manoeuvre (manipulation of a guidewire). In this case, the catheter is treated by advancing a guide wire out of the end of the CVC in the hope of dislodging a small thrombus or moving the catheter tip to a more favourable location. The effect of deflecting the tip of the a tunnelled line is likely only temporary. Also, creating a 0.035 hole through an occlusive thrombus or fibrin sheath at the catheter tip is unlikely to provide an adequate lumen for dialysis. Moving the catheter tip or the entire catheter with a guidewire is difficult because the subcutaneous cuff is not released [61] (Fig. 8.15).

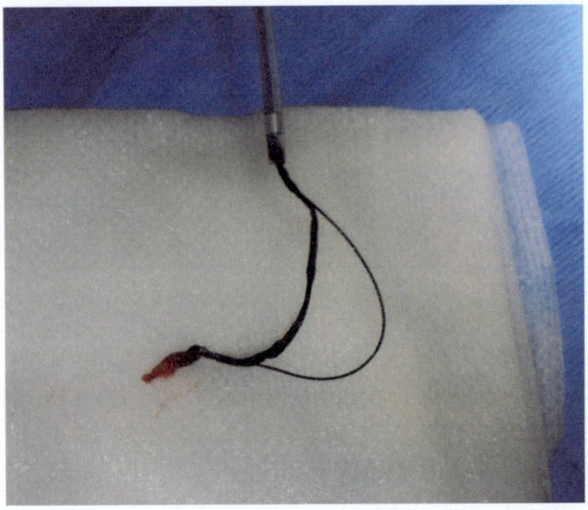

Fig. 8.14 Fibrin sheath removal with loop snare. (Dr Federica Ferro, Interventional Radiology, Bolzano Hospital, Italy)

Fully Implantable Haemodialysis Systems

Special dual-chamber venous ports for haemodialysis were also attempted in the past. However, they have today been almost completely dismissed because they are not cost-effective [62].

Paediatric Haemodialysis Access

In the choice of the vein, the same considerations apply to adult patients, where supraclavicular veins (anonymous or jugular) are preferred over axillary veins. Atrial tip placement prevents occlusions due to the vessel wall and allows efficient dialysis. Femoral access should be reserved for cases where upper-body venous access is no longer available. A 3–5 mL/kg/min flow is acceptable in most patients. The appropriate size of a tunnelled or non-tunnelled, cuffed CVC in paediatric patients ranges from 6.0 to 7.0 Fr for patients weighing less than 10 kg, 6.0–8.0 Fr for patients weighing between 10 and 30 kg, 8.0–10.0 Fr for patients weighing between 30 and 50 kg, and 11.5 Fr or more for children weighing more than 50 kg [58] (Table 8.4).

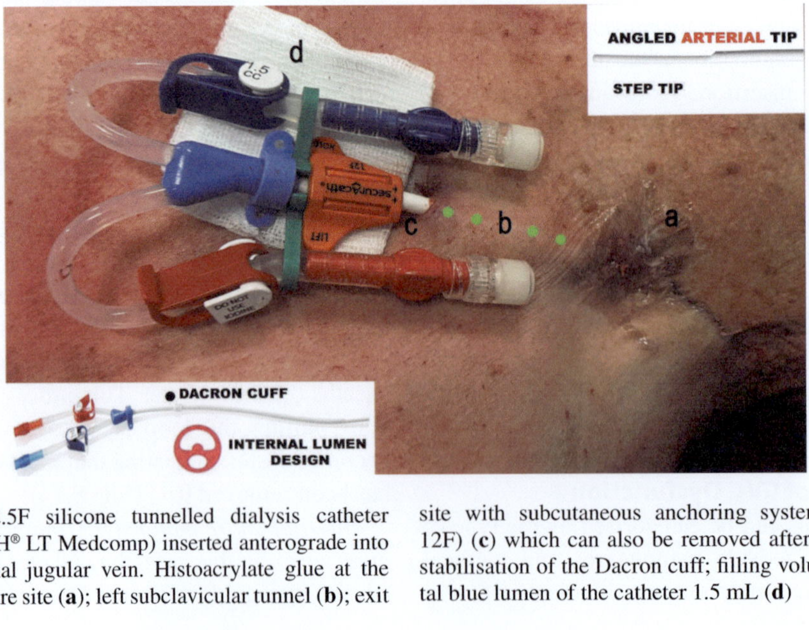

Fig. 8.15 12.5F silicone tunnelled dialysis catheter (HEMO-CATH® LT Medcomp) inserted anterograde into the left internal jugular vein. Histoacrylate glue at the venous puncture site (**a**); left subclavicular tunnel (**b**); exit site with subcutaneous anchoring system (Securacath 12F) (**c**) which can also be removed after 3 weeks after stabilisation of the Dacron cuff; filling volume of the distal blue lumen of the catheter 1.5 mL (**d**)

Table 8.4 Summary of characteristics of long-term, cuffed dialysis central venous catheter

Venous access of choice	Like short-term
Tip location	Like short-term
Duration	There is no maximum time limit to CVC use, but regular evaluation is required to determine if the CVC remains the most appropriate dialysis access
Management	Like short-term

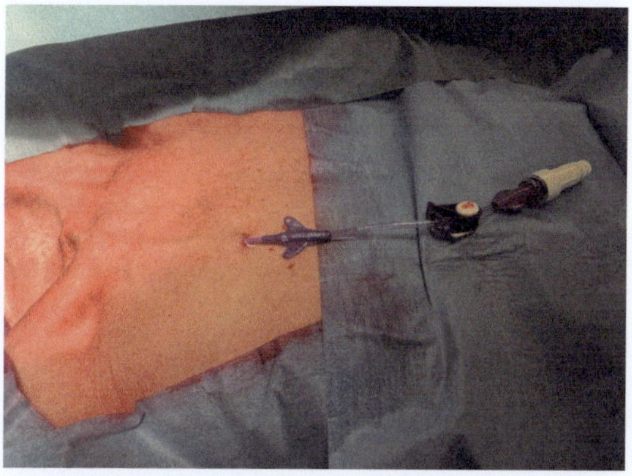

Fig. 8.16 Small-bore cuffed tunnelled catheter (Pro-Line®—Medcomp, 5F power) inserted in the right internal jugular vein and tunnelled with exit site on the right side of the chest

Central Venous Access in the Nephropathic Patient for Diseases Unrelated to Renal Failure

Any central and peripheral venous access can compromise the patient's venous patrimony, whether in acute or chronic situations. In patients with renal failure in particular, venous access should be oriented to vein routes that may not compromise the confection of an arteriovenous fistula or the availability of iliac vessels for possible renal transplantation.

Patients in chronic or impending renal failure may need central venous access for issues unrelated to renal failure. PICCs would provide safe and cost-effective central venous access in hospitalised and home-treated patients. However, preserving central and peripheral venous supply in this patient population requires a different strategy when choosing venous access than in other patients.

In patients with stage 4–5 acute renal failure, forearm and arm veins that might be suitable for fistula creation, subclavian-axillary catheters, or PICCs should not be used for cannulation due to the risk of central venous stenosis and occlusion [56, 60].

In conclusion, the logical choice for a nephropathic patient requiring temporary central venous access is to use the anonymous or internal jugular vein. Some authors have also proposed tunnelling temporary accesses in these patients to minimise the infectious risk [63].

Infectiologists' guidelines encourage PICC implantation for intravenous antibiotic therapy, while nephrologists' guidelines discourage it in CKI patients. The best-known alternatives to PICCs are large-calibre tunnelled catheters. However, options for small-diameter PICCs (small-diameter tunnelled CICCs), which have few complications and nonsymptomatic central thrombosis or stenosis and avoid cannulation of the cephalic and basilic veins used to create fistulas, are not well known [64] (Fig. 8.16).

References

1. Kehagias E, Galanakis N, Tsetis D. Central venous catheters: which, when and how. Br J Radiol. 2023;96(1151):20220894.
2. Khwaja A. KDIGO clinical practice guidelines for acute kidney injury. Nephron Clin Pract. 2012;120(4):c179–84.
3. O'Grady NP, Alexander M, Burns LA, Dellinger EP, Garland J, Heard SO, et al. Guidelines for the prevention of intravascular catheter-related infections. Am J Infect Control. 2011;39(4 Suppl 1):S1–34.
4. Parienti JJ, Mongardon N, Megarbane B, Mira JP, Kalfon P, Gros A, et al. Intravascular complications of central venous catheterization by insertion site. N Engl J Med. 2015;373(13):1220–9.
5. Practice guidelines for central venous access 2020: an updated report by the American Society of Anesthesiologists Task Force on Central Venous Access. Anesthesiology. 2020;132(1):8–43.
6. Brass P, Hellmich M, Kolodziej L, Schick G, Smith AF. Ultrasound guidance versus anatomical landmarks for internal jugular vein catheterization. Cochrane Database Syst Rev. 2015;1(1):CD006962.

7. Safety Committee of Japanese Society of Anesthesiologists. Practical guide for safe central venous catheterization and management 2017. J Anesth. 2020;34(2):167–86.
8. Yu C, Shulan L, Juan W, Ling L, Chun-Mei L. The accuracy and safety of using the electrocardiogram positioning technique in localizing the peripherally inserted central catheter tip position: a systematic review and meta-analysis. Nurs Open. 2022;9(3):1556–63.
9. Bannon MP, Heller SF, Rivera M. Anatomic considerations for central venous cannulation. Risk Manag Healthc Policy. 2011;4:27–39.
10. Mumtaz S, Singh M. Surgical review of the anatomical variations of the internal jugular vein: an update for head and neck surgeons. Ann R Coll Surg Engl. 2019;101(1):2–6.
11. Ge X, Cavallazzi R, Li C, Pan SM, Wang YW, Wang FL. Central venous access sites for the prevention of venous thrombosis, stenosis and infection. Cochrane Database Syst Rev. 2012;2012(3):CD004084.
12. Timsit JF, Bouadma L, Mimoz O, Parienti JJ, Garrouste-Orgeas M, Alfandari S, et al. Jugular versus femoral short-term catheterization and risk of infection in intensive care unit patients. Causal analysis of two randomized trials. Am J Respir Crit Care Med. 2013;188(10):1232–9.
13. Kapoor MC. Alternative approaches to central venous cannulation in cardiac surgery. Ann Card Anaesth. 2023;26(4):365–6.
14. Krishnan AK, Menon P, Gireesh Kumar KP, Sreekrishnan TP, Garg M, Kumar SV. Electrocardiogram-guided technique: an alternative method for confirming central venous catheter tip placement. J Emerg Trauma Shock. 2018;11(4):276–81.
15. Winkler M, Talley C, Woodward C, et al. The use of intraosseous needles for injection of contrast media for computed tomographic angiography of the thoracic aorta. J Cardiovasc Comput Tomogr. 2017;11(3):203–7.
16. Lewis P, Wright C. Saving the critically injured trauma patient: a retrospective analysis of 1000 uses of intraosseous access. Emerg Med J. 2014;32(6):463–7.
17. Hamed RK, Hartmans S, Gausche-Hill M. Anesthesia through an intraosseous line using an 18-gauge intravenous needle for emergency pediatric surgery. J Clin Anesth. 2013;25(6):447–51.
18. Aliman AC, Piccioni Mde A, Piccioni JL, Oliva JL, Auler Junior JO. Intraosseous anesthesia in hemodynamic studies in children with cardiopathy. Rev Bras Anestesiol. 2011;61(1):41–9.
19. Loughren M, Banks S, Naluan C, Portenlanger P, Wendorf A, Johnson D. Onset and duration of intravenous and intraosseous rocuronium in swine. West J Emerg Med. 2014;XV(2):241–5.
20. Barnard EB, Moy RJ, Kehoe AD, Bebarta TS, Smith JE. Rapid sequence induction of anesthesia via the intraosseous route: a prospective observational study. Emerg Med J. 2015;32(6):449–52.
21. Bebarta TS, Vargas TE, Castaneda M, Boudreau S. Evaluation of extremity tissue and bone injury after intraosseous hypertonic saline infusion in proximal tibia and proximal humerus in adult swine. Prehosp Emerg Care. 2014;18(4):505–10.
22. Schlimp CJ, Solomon C, Keibl C, et al. Recovery of fibrinogen concentrate after intraosseous application is equivalent to the intravenous route in a porcine model of hemodilution. J Trauma Acute Care Surg. 2014;76(5):1235–42.
23. Spencer TR. Intraosseous administration of thrombolytics for pulmonary embolism. J Emerg Med. 2013;45(6):197–200.
24. Johnson D, Dial J, Ard J, et al. Effects of intraosseous and intravenous administration of Hextend on time of administration and hemodynamics in a swine model. J Spec Oper Med. 2014;14(1):79–85.
25. Chansa E, Kansen K, Gustafsson B. An intraosseous blood transfusion in a critically ill child [Une transfusion sanguine par voie intraosseuse chez un enfant gravement malade]. Afr J Emerg Med. 2013;4:83. https://doi.org/10.1016/j.afjem.2013.05.003.
26. Anson JA. Vascular access in resuscitation: is there a role for the intraosseous route? Anesthesiology. 2014;120(4):1015–31.
27. Anson JA, Sinz EH, Swick JT. The versatility of intraosseous vascular access in perioperative medicine: a case series. J Clin Anesth. 2015;27(1):63–7.
28. Frascone RJ, Salzman JG, Bliss P, Adams A, Wewerka SS, Dries DJ. Intraosseous pressure tracings mimic arterial pressure tracings in timing and contour. Ann Emerg Med. 2013;62(4s):s13.
29. Von Hoff DD, Kuhn JG, Burris HA, Miller LJ. Does intraosseous equal intravenous? A pharmacokinetic study. Am J Emerg Med. 2008;26:31–8.
30. Montez DF, Puga T, Miller L, et al. Intraosseous infusions from the proximal humerus reach the heart in less than 3 seconds in human volunteers. Ann Emerg Med. 2015;66(4):S47.
31. Frascone RJ, Salzman JG, Adams AB, Bliss P, Wewerka SS, Dries DJ. Evaluation of intraosseous pressure in a hypovolemic animal model. J Surg Res. 2015;193:383–90.
32. Salzman JG, Frascone RJ, Zagar AE, et al. Intraosseous pressure monitoring in critical care patients. Ann Emerg Med. 2015;66(4s):S148.
33. American Heart Association. 2010 American Heart Association guidelines for CPR and ECC. Part 14 – Pediatric advanced life support. Circulation. 2010;122(3 suppl):S881–5.
34. Monsieurs KG, Nolan JP, Bossaert LL, et al. European Resuscitation Council guidelines for resuscitation 2015. Resuscitation. 2015;95:1–80.
35. Gorski L, Hadaway L, Hagle ME, et al. Infusion therapy standards of practice. J Infus Nurs. 2016;39(1S):S1–S159. ISSN 1533-1458. www.journalofinfusionnursing.com.
36. Jousi M, Björkman J, Nurmi J. Point-of-care analyses of blood samples from intraosseous access in pre-hospital critical care. Acta Anaesthesiol Scand.

2019;63:1419. https://doi.org/10.1111/aas.13443. [Epub ahead of print]
37. Lewis P, Wright C. Saving the critically injured trauma patient: a retrospective analysis of 1000 uses of intraosseous access. Emerg J Med. 2010;39(4):468–75.
38. Jousi M, Laukkanen-Nevala P, Nurmi J. Analysing blood from intraosseous access: a systemic review. Eur J Emerg Med. 2019;26(2):77–85.
39. Greenstein YY, Koenig SJ, Mayo PH, Narasimhan M. A serious adult intraosseous catheter complication and review of the literature. Crit Care Med. 2016;44(9):e904–9.
40. Petitpas F, Guenezan J, Vendeuvre T, Scepi M, Oriot D, Mimoz O. Use of intraosseous access in adults: a systematic review. Crit Care. 2016;20:102.
41. Rubal BJ, Meyers BL, Kramer SA, Hanson MA, Andrews JM, DeLorenzo RA. Fat intravasation from intraosseous flush and infusion procedures. Prehosp Emerg Care. 2015;19(3):376–90.
42. D'Onofrio G, Zini G. Analysis of bone marrow aspiration fluid using automated blood cell counters. Clin Lab Med. 2015;35(1):25–42.
43. Ginsberg-Peltz J. Time to bone healing after intraosseous placement in children is ill defined. Pediatr Emerg Care. 2016;32(11):799–800.
44. Voigt J, Waltzman M, Lottenberg L. Intraosseous vascular access for in-hospital emergency use: a systematic clinical review of the literature and analysis. Pediatr Emerg Care. 2012;28(2):185–998.
45. Neumar RW, Otto CW, Link MS, et al. Adult advanced cardiovascular life support. 2010 American Heart Association guidelines for Cardiopulmonary Resuscitation and Emergency Cardiovascular Care. Circulation. 2010;122(suppl 3):S729–67.
46. Bartl R, Bartl C. Evolution of the skeleton. In: The osteoporosis manual. Cham: Springer; 2019. https://doi.org/10.1007/978-3-030-00731-7_1.
47. Quibell K, Yip J. Intraosseous access site selection. In: Paxton JH, editor. Intraosseous vascular access. Cham: Springer; 2024. https://doi.org/10.1007/978-3-031-61201-5_4.
48. Philbeck TE, Miller LJ, Montez D, Puga T. Hurts so good; easing IO pain and pressure. JEMS. 2010;35(9):58–69.
49. Philbeck TE, Puga T, Montez DF, Miller LJ, Saussy J, Davlantes C. Sternal flow rates and insertion success using a multisite intraosseous device. Ann Emerg Med. 2015;66(4s):S48.
50. Puga T, Montez D, Philbeck T, Davlantes C. Adequacy of intraosseous vascular access insertion sites for high-volume fluid infusion. Crit Care Med. 2016;44(12):143.
51. Davlantes C, Puga T, Montez D, Philbeck T, Miller L, DeNoia E. 48 hours dwell time for intraosseous access: a longer-term infusion using a temporary solution. Crit Care Med. 2016;44(12):140.TS.
52. Montez D, Puga T, Davlantes C, Philbeck T. IO infusion pain mitigation in the sternum and proximal humerus: establishing a regimen. Crit Care Med. 2016;44(12):154.
53. Patel NH, Revanur VK, Khanna A, Hodges C, Jindal RM. Vascular access for hemodialysis: an indepth review. J Nephrol. 2001;14(3):146–56.
54. Trerotola SO. Hemodialysis catheter placement and management. Radiology. 2000;215(3):651–8.
55. Aitken DR, Minton JP. The pinch-off sign: a warning of impending problems with permanent subclavian catheters. Am J Surg. 1984;148:633–8.
56. National Kidney Foundation. Guideline 2. Selection and placement of hemodialysis access. In: 2006 Updates clinical practice guidelines and recommendations. NKF; 2006.
57. Nickel B, Gorski L, Kleidon T, et al. Infusion therapy standards of practice. J Infus Nurs. 2024;47(1S):S1–S285.
58. Lok CE, Huber TS, Lee T, Shenoy S, Yevzlin AS, Abreo K, Allon M, Asif A, Astor BC, Glickman MH, Graham J, Moist LM, Rajan DK, Roberts C, Vachharajani TJ, Valentini RP, National Kidney Foundation. KDOQI clinical practice guideline for vascular access: 2019 update. Am J Kidney Dis. 2020;75(4 Suppl 2):S1–S164.
59. Schindler R. Vaskulärer Zugang für die Nierenersatztherapie. In: Jörres A, Hrsg. Akutes Nierenversagen bei Intensivpatienten – Praxis und Therapie. Köln: Deutscher Ärzte Verlag; 2010.
60. Gorski LA, Hadaway L, Hagle ME, et al. Infusion therapy standards of practice. J Infus Nurs. 2021;44(1S):S1–S224.
61. Angle JF, Shilling AT, Schenk WG, Bissonette EA, Stadtlander KS, Hagspiel KD, Spinosa DJ, Leung DA, Matsumoto AH. Utility of percutaneous intervention in the management of tunneled hemodialysis catheters. Cardiovasc Intervent Radiol. 2003;26:9–18.
62. Canaud B, My H, Morena M, Lamy-Lacavalerie B, Leray-Moragues H, Bosc JY, Flavier JL, Chomel PY, Polaschegg HD, Prosl FR, Megerman J. Dialock: a new vascular access device for extracorporeal renal replacement therapy. Preliminary clinical results. Nephrol Dial Transplant. 1999;14(3):692–8.
63. Sasadeusz KJ, Trerotola SO, Shah H, Namyslowski J, Johnson MS, Moresco KP, Patel NH. Tunneled jugular small-bore central catheters as an alternative to peripherally inserted central catheters for intermediate-term venous access in patients with hemodialysis and chronic renal insufficiency. Radiology. 1999;213(1):303–6.
64. Chopra V, Flanders SA, Saint S, Woller SC, O'Grady NP, Safdar N, Trerotola SO, Saran R, Moureau N, Wiseman S, Pittiruti M, Akl EA, Lee AY, Courey A, Swaminathan L, LeDonne J, Becker C, Krein SL, Bernstein SJ, Michigan Appropriateness Guide for Intravenouse Catheters (MAGIC) Panel. The Michigan Appropriateness Guide for Intravenous Catheters (MAGIC): results from a multispecialty panel using the RAND/UCLA appropriateness method. Ann Intern Med. 2015;163(6):S1–S39.

9 Future Directions and Advances

Massimo Lamperti

The increasing use of ultrasound (US) has been pivotal in reducing many of the mechanical complications related to the insertion of central venous lines, but some technical issues (e.g. alignment of the needle entry with the target vessel) still prevent the rate of complications from being completely zero. Central line-associated bloodstream infection (CLABSI) is another critical problem, and many efforts have been made to reduce this life-threatening hospital-acquired infection (HAI). A standardised education is also needed to train future generations of clinicians on why a central line is required and how it has to be placed and maintained.

Emerging Technologies and Techniques for Central Venous Cannulation

Performing central venous catheterisation (CVC) can be particularly challenging in deep anatomical sites, such as the subclavian vein, and in patients with certain conditions, such as obesity or a history of local surgery. New real-time ultrasound-guided technologies have been developed to address these difficulties and improve the procedure's comfort and safety. These advancements allow for better visualisation of anatomical structures, facilitating more accurate needle placement and reducing the risk of complications.

Magnetic Devices

Magnetic devices enhance real-time visualisation of the needle and its precise location relative to the ultrasound beam, potentially improving success rates and reducing complications. A recent randomised controlled simulation study evaluated the efficacy and safety of axillary/subclavian vein catheterisation using a novel magnetic needle-pilot system compared to traditional ultrasound guidance [1]. The needle-pilot device improved the time to successful cannulation (22 s (interquartile range (IQR) = 16–42) vs. 25 s (IQR = 19–128); median of difference (MOD) = −9 s (95% confidence interval (CI) −5, −22); $p < 0.001$). The rates of skin punctures, posterior wall puncture of the axillary vein, and needle redirections were also lower ($p < 0.01$). Comfort was higher in the needle-pilot US-guided group on an 11-point numeric scale (8 (IQR = 8–9) vs. 6 (IQR = 6–8); $p < 0.001$). While these promising results were observed on a simulation mannequin, they need to be validated by a randomised controlled trial (RCT) in intensive care patients.

M. Lamperti (✉)
Anesthesiology Division, Cleveland Clinic
Abu Dhabi, Abu Dhabi, UAE

R. Lanocita, M. Lamperti (eds.), *Practical Guide to Central Venous Cannulation*,
https://doi.org/10.1007/978-3-031-90326-7_9

Specific Needles

New photoacoustic needles represent a promising technology based on innovative principles. An optical fibre is inserted into the lumen of a standard needle without occlusion, transmitting pulsed laser light from an external source. This light is then converted into ultrasound waves, which the ultrasound probe receives for imaging [2]. A pilot study demonstrated a significantly improved ability to identify the needle tip on recorded videos [2]. Further research is needed to evaluate the effectiveness of this promising technology in clinical practice.

Despite the use of ultrasound guidance for internal jugular vein (IJV) cannulation, studies using human simulators have reported a puncture incidence of approximately 20% for the carotid artery and 64% for the posterior venous wall. A recent study by Arya and colleagues [3] devised a guard which can be slid and fixed over the needle at a desired length (measured through ultrasound), thus preventing the needle from penetrating deeper into the skin beyond this guard (Fig. 9.1).

A total of 419 patients were randomised into control ($n = 209$) and study ($n = 210$) groups. The study group had a significantly higher rate of successful IJV cannulation on the first attempt (primary endpoint) than the control group (98.6% vs. 85.7%; $p = 0.007$). Posterior venous wall puncture occurred in 0.5% (1/210) of the study group versus 8.61% (18/209) of the control group ($p = 0.001$). Common carotid artery puncture was 7.18% (15/209) in the control group and 0% (0/210) in the study group ($p = 0.001$). Operators reported significantly better ease of use in the study group ($p < 0.001$).

Smart Glasses

Successful ultrasound-guided vascular access requires anatomical knowledge and coordination between hands, eyes, the procedure field, and the ultrasound screen. During the procedure, frequent head and eye movements are needed to align the target vessel, ultrasound probe, and needle tip. These movements can increase procedure time, disrupt the grip on the ultrasound probe, potentially lose the target vessel image, and lead to incorrect needle direction.

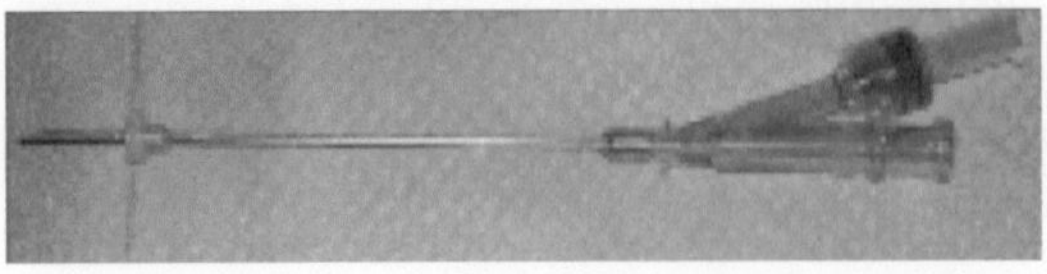

Fig. 9.1 Puncture needle with guard

Recently, head-mounted displays like smart glasses have gained popularity in medical practice. When connected to an ultrasound machine, smart glasses project the ultrasound screen directly in front of the operator's eyes, allowing simultaneous visualisation of both the procedure field and the ultrasound screen without requiring head and eye movements. Studies have demonstrated the impact of head-mounted displays on reducing head and neck movement during adult vascular access using central venous catheterisation simulators and peripheral vascular phantoms [4, 5].

A randomised controlled trial enrolled paediatric patients ($n = 116$, age less than 2 years) requiring radial artery cannulation during general anaesthesia (Fig. 9.2).

The participants were randomised into the ultrasound screen group (control) or the smart glasses group. The smart glasses group demonstrated a higher first-attempt success rate than the control group (87.9% vs. 72.4%; $p = 0.036$). The procedure time for the first attempt was significantly shorter in the smart glasses group (median, 33 s; interquartile range (IQR), 23–47 s; range, 10–141 s) than in the control group (median, 43 s; IQR 31–67 s; range, 17–248 s; $p = 0.007$). The smart glasses group also had a lower overall complication rate (5.2% [3/58] vs. 29.3%; $p = 0.001$). Additionally, the proportion of positive ergonomic satisfaction (ratings of 4 = good or 5 = best) was significantly higher in the smart glasses group (65.5% vs. 20.7%; $p < 0.001$).

A simulation study using a phantom model [6] revealed a 17% improvement in procedure time for novices, while experienced participants saw a 5% increase in duration, potentially indicating a bias due to their extensive training and experience. This technique has yet to be evaluated for central venous catheterisation (CVC) in intensive care patients.

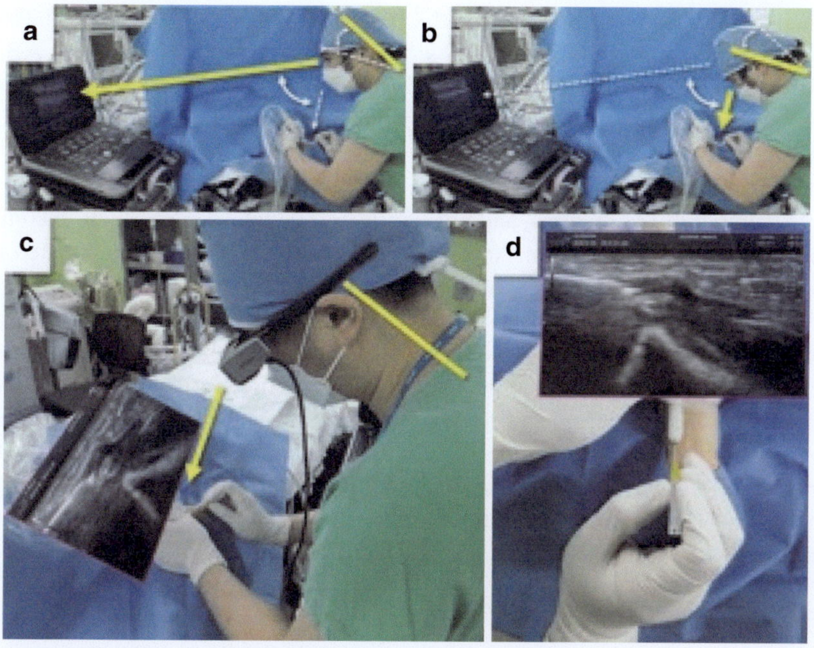

Fig. 9.2 Ultrasound-guided radial artery cannulation in the control group (**a**, **b**) and the smart glasses group (**c**, **d**). The thick yellow lines indicate the operator's cervical spine and gaze, and the thin white lines and arrows indicate the range of motion. (**a**) The operator is looking at the ultrasound screen to find the radial artery. (**b**) The operator moved his head, neck, and eyes to look at the procedure field (cannulation site). (**c**) With smart glasses, the operator can focus on the ultrasound screen and procedure field (cannulation site) simultaneously without moving his head. (**d**) Real-time ultrasound screen by smart glasses over the procedure field in the operator's view. (From: Jang et al. [30])

3D Biplane Technologies

3D ultrasound probes provide detailed and comprehensive images of anatomical structures, offering a clearer and more accurate view than traditional 2D imaging. This can be particularly beneficial for allowing short- and long-axis visualisation simultaneously. The literature has contradictory evidence on their use in central line catheterisation.

A non-randomised prospective study from Panidapu [7] was divided into two groups of 50 (biplanar group (BPX) and short-axis (SAX) group) by assigning the study participants alternatively to each group. An experienced anaesthesiologist performed IJV cannulation using a 3D ultrasound probe in all patients with either the BPX view (BPX group, $n = 50$) or the SAX view (SAX group, $n = 50$). The time taken for imaging was significantly greater in the BPX group than in the SAX group (9.52 ± 2.69 s vs. 7.94 ± 2.55 s; $p = 0.0034$), whereas the time taken for IJV puncture (10.39 ± 2.33 s vs. 23.7 ± 2.46 s; $p < 0.0001$), time taken for confirmation of guidewire (32.94 ± 4.50 s vs. 57.64 ± 7.14 s; $p < 0.0001$), and the incidence of posterior wall puncture (4% vs. 26%; $p = 0.0022$) were significantly less in the BPX group than in the SAX group. The total number of attempts taken to puncture the IJV was fewer in the BPX group than in the SAX group (55 vs. 78). Successful puncture of the IJV occurred on the first attempt in 90% of patients in the BPX group, whereas it was only 50% in the SAX group ($p < 0.0001$). The quality of needle visualisation was good in 90% of patients in the BPX group, whereas it was only 6% in the SAX group. The number of needle redirections for IJV puncture was less in the BPX group than in the SAX group (48 vs. 116). The incidence of complications was not significant between the two groups.

These favourable results were not confirmed by a recent RCT [8] in simulated central line placement by emergency physicians in which the short-axis imaged approach was associated with a significantly shorter time to cannulation (34.9 s vs. 17.6; $p < 0.001$) and time to scout (30 vs. 49 s; $p = 0.008$) when compared to biplane-axis imaging approach. No significant differences were noted when comparing first-pass success, number of attempts, number of redirections, and posterior wall and arterial wall puncture. Another RCT on IJV catheterisation [9] did not show any significant difference in first-pass success without withdrawals (72.1% and 75.4%; $p = 0.68$) or within one skin break (90.2% and 90.8%; $p = 0.58$) in the 2D and 3D groups, respectively. Scanning and procedure times were longer, and subjective mental effort was higher using 3D guidance. There was a trend towards more posterior wall punctures without carotid artery punctures for 3D imaging.

Research on Reducing Complications and Improving Patient Outcomes

Short-term central venous catheters (CVCs) are vital for diagnosing and treating of hospitalised patients with the most diverse clinical conditions [10]. However, the rate of complications associated with the insertion procedure is high. It is a significant cause of preventable morbidity and mortality [11]. The use of the subclavian vein is more related to pneumothorax and less to infections, and the internal jugular and femoral veins are more related to arterial perforation [12]. The CLABSI rates reported by the World Health Organization, through a systematic review and meta-analysis of published data, identified that in high-income countries, the CLABSI rate was 3.5 CLABSI per 1000 CL-days, while in low- and middle-income countries (LMICs), it was 12.2 [13]. CLABSIs have a significant impact on healthcare, leading to increased mortality rates [14, 15], with CLABSIs associated with a 12–25% increase in mortality [15]. Pooling 630 ICUs from 2015 to 2020 of 45 LMICs, the mortality rates were as follows: 14.06% for patients without HAI and 39.81% for those with CLABSI. Patients with two simultaneous HAIs experienced mortality rates ranging from 38.79% to 43.32%, while those with all three types of HAIs (CLABSI + ventilator-associated pneumonia (VAP) + catheter-associated urinary tract infection (CAUTI)) had a mortality rate of 46.56%.

From 1998 to 2022, a multinational, multicentre prospective cohort study encompassing 728 ICUs within 286 hospitals situated in 147 cities across 41 African, Asian, Eastern European, Latin American, and Middle Eastern countries, utilising an online standardised surveillance system and unified forms, identified factors independently associated with CLABSI, including a 3% daily risk increase in CLABSI with prolonged LOS ($p < 0.0001$), a 4% risk increase per CL-day ($p < 0.0001$), surgical hospitalisation ($p < 0.0001$), tracheostomy use ($p < 0.0001$), hospitalisation at a publicly owned facility ($p < 0.0001$) or at a teaching hospital ($p < 0.0001$), and hospitalisation in a middle-income country ($p < 0.0001$), with the highest CLABSI risk observed in adult oncology ($p < 0.0001$), followed by paediatric oncology ($p < 0.0001$), and PICU ($p < 0.0001$), while the highest CLABSI risk was associated with internal jugular ($p < 0.0001$), followed by femoral ($p < 0.0001$), and the lowest CLABSI risk was found with PICCs ($p = 0.04$) [16].

The Recommendations for The Prevention of Central Line-Associated Bloodstream Infections from the International Society for Infectious Disease [17] and the Strategies to prevent central line-associated bloodstream infections in acute-care hospitals: 2022 Update sponsored by the Society for Healthcare Epidemiology of America (SHEA) [18] are summarised in Table 9.1 with all the practical recommendations to assist acute-care hospitals in implementing and prioritising their central line-associated bloodstream infection (CLABSI) prevention efforts.

Prevention of CLABSI depends on integrating best practices to reduce the risk of infection and incorporating a culture to support implementation. Hospitals should address technical and socio-adaptive components [19] to CLABSI prevention, including formal training of healthcare providers on indications, placement, and maintenance of devices and regular assessment of competencies [20].

Table 9.1 Summary of SEHA recommendations (adapted from Buetti et al. [18]) and level of evidence (LoE)

Essential practices
Before insertion
1. Provide easy access to an evidence-based list of indications for CVC use to minimise unnecessary CVC placement (LoE low)
2. Require education and competency assessment of healthcare personnel involved in insertion, care, and maintenance of CVCs about CLABSI prevention (LoE moderate)
3. Bathe ICU patients aged >2 months with a chlorhexidine preparation on a daily basis (LoE high)
At insertion
1. In ICU and non-ICU settings, a facility should have a process in place, such as a checklist, to ensure adherence to infection prevention practices at the time of CVC insertion (LoE moderate)
2. Perform hand hygiene prior to catheter insertion or manipulation (LoE moderate)
3. The subclavian site is preferred to reduce infectious complications when the catheter is placed in the ICU setting(LoE high)
4. Use an all-inclusive catheter cart or kit (LoE moderate)
5. Use ultrasound guidance for catheter insertion (LoE high)
6. Use maximum sterile barrier precautions during CVC insertion (LoE moderate)
7. Use an alcoholic chlorhexidine antiseptic for skin preparation (LoE high)
After insertion
1. Ensure appropriate nurse-to-patient ratio and limit use of float nurses in ICUs (LoE high)
2. Use chlorhexidine-containing dressings for CVCs in patients over 2 months of age (LoE high)
3. For non-tunnelled CVCs in adults and children, change transparent dressings and perform site care with a chlorhexidine-based antiseptic at least every 7 days or immediately if the dressing is soiled, loose, or damp. Change gauze dressings every 2 days or earlier if the dressing is soiled, loose, or damp (LoE moderate)
4. Disinfect catheter hubs, needleless connectors, and injection ports before accessing the catheter (LoE moderate)
5. Remove nonessential catheters (LoE moderate)
6. Routine replacement of administration sets not used for blood, blood products, or lipid formulations can be performed at intervals up to 7 days (LoE high)
7. Perform surveillance for CLABSI in ICU and non-ICU settings (LoE high)
Additional approaches
1. Use antiseptic- or antimicrobial-impregnated CVCs (LoE high in adults and moderate in paediatrics)
2. Use antimicrobial lock therapy for long-term CVCs (LoE high)
3. Use recombinant tissue plasminogen activating factor (rt-PA) once weekly after haemodialysis in patients undergoing haemodialysis through a CVC (LoE high)
4. Utilise infusion or vascular access teams for reducing CLABSI rates (LoE low)
5. Use antimicrobial ointments for haemodialysis catheter insertion sites (LoE high)
6. Use an antiseptic-containing hub/connector cap/port protector to cover connectors (LoE moderate)
Approaches that should not be considered a routine part of CLABSI prevention
1. Do not use antimicrobial prophylaxis for short-term or tunnelled catheter insertion or while catheters are in situ (LoE high)
2. Do not routinely replace CVCs or arterial catheters (LoE high)
Unresolved issues
1. Routine use of needleless connectors as a CLABSI prevention strategy before an assessment of risks, benefits, and education regarding proper use
2. Surveillance of other types of catheters (e.g., peripheral arterial or peripheral venous catheters)
3. Standard, nonantimicrobial transparent dressings and CLABSI risk
4. The impact of using chlorhexidine-based products on bacterial resistance to chlorhexidine
5. Sutureless securement
6. Impact of silver zeolite-impregnated umbilical catheters in preterm infants (applicable in countries where it is approved for use in children)
7. Necessity of mechanical disinfection of a catheter hub, needleless connector, and injection port before accessing the catheter when antiseptic-containing caps are being used

One example of a widely used model in the United States, known as the four Es (i.e. engage, educate, execute, and evaluate) [21], summarised in Table 9.2, involves summarising evidence, identifying local barriers to implementation, measuring performance, and ensuring that patients receive the infection prevention intervention [22] by addressing knowledge, critical

Table 9.2 The four Es concept in CLABSI prevention

Engage
Having a frontline and leadership champions to support CLABSI reduction initiatives. Champions are often very effective in initial phases of adoption, but their efforts should aim to be long-lasting
Educate
1. Appropriate indications prior to insertion 2. Use of full barrier precautions at the time of insertion 3. Daily evaluation of necessity of the device
Execute
A standardised competency assessment checklist should be used to assess and document competency of each individual performing CVC insertion and procedures related to care and maintenance (e.g. dressing changes)
Evaluate
• Multidisciplinary teams should set clear goals and identify the key factors to be measured. It is important for members of the healthcare team to receive feedback on their performance. Feedback should include periodic (e.g. monthly and quarterly) communication (e.g. e-mail messages and written reports) of process measurement data via posters, reports, or other forms of communication with graphs showing cumulative compliance with process measures • Differences between age groups should also be considered (e.g. neonates, paediatrics, and adults) • Central line data can be used to capture trends over time. The standardised utilisation ratio (SUR) provides a method for the hospital's units to compare themselves to others with similar characteristics. CLABSI events are important to discuss with the different members of the team caring for the patient to have a clear understanding of gaps and ways to mitigate them in the future

thinking, behaviour and psychomotor skills, and attitudes and beliefs of all members of the healthcare team involved with the insertion and care of CVCs.

CLABSI still ranks as the main fatal complication related to a central venous catheter. While further research is still needed in some areas, the key to reducing complications is full adherence to bundles and evidence-based recommendations frequently not followed in clinical practice.

Training and Education for Clinicians Performing Central Venous Cannulation

Safe central venous catheterisation and management require standardised education, simulations, and well-defined instructional frameworks [23].

Ultrasound guidance has been recognised as the safest technique for most central venous accesses [24], but training in all techniques, including ultrasound assistance, is still part of the training of novices approaching this procedure.

To master this skill, simulation training has proven effective [25–27]; however, it is unclear whether simulation-based education actually reduces the incidence of adverse events. Fine control of the needle tip is probably necessary to prevent adverse events. Simulation-based education might be required for outcome-based task training. Institutions and hospitals should incorporate mannequins and other educational tools for puncture simulations. If acquiring such equipment independently is challenging, joint training sessions at academic conferences or similar events are recommended. These sessions can also teach rapid complication detection techniques. Additionally, simulation training should include infection control practices [28].

Simulation training on cadavers for high-risk procedures has recently become feasible and has shown some effectiveness [29]. We recommend that novice operators undergo cadaver training at the beginning of their clinical training, guided by experts and educational specialists.

Training programmes should focus on improving technical skills and covering safety protocols, infection control, informed consent procedures, and communication skills.

The evidence-based consensus on the insertion of central venous access devices: definition of minimal requirements for training by Moureau and colleagues [23] summarised the different components of training in central vascular access, focusing on the minimal level of education required for safe insertion procedures and management of central venous access devices (CVADs).

Clinicians involved in placing CVADs with ultrasound guidance need proper education and training to ensure patient safety and avoid major complications during the insertion process. Standard didactic education should include basic knowledge of anatomy, ultrasound physics and imaging, and infection prevention strategies. These topics are essential for a thorough understanding and safe execution of the insertion procedure.

Learning Methods

There are different methods for teaching adults new concepts or practical skills:

1. Experiential education is a methodology where educators and mentors engage learners in direct experience and reflection to enhance knowledge, develop skills, and clarify values. This method must consider the learner's prior experience, knowledge base, and theoretical preparation. The context of learning will vary, but it generally guides learners from being dependent to becoming supervised participants and ultimately achieving supported independence.
2. Situated learning is a model where learning occurs through active or guided participation within a community of practice. This model emphasises that students learn best when involved in authentic professional activities supported by experienced and capable mentors. Guided participation, a key component of situated learning, involves several elements:
   - Cognitive ability: Engaging in thinking processes
   - Problem-solving: Developing skills to address and resolve real-world challenges
   - Adequate knowledge: Acquiring necessary information relevant to the practice
   - Personal skills: Cultivating interpersonal and professional skills
   - Appropriate attitudes and values: Adopting the right mindset and ethical standards

   The role of the mentor is crucial in this model. The mentor, an experienced practitioner, acts as the most valuable resource for the learner, providing support, guidance, and insights drawn from their professional experiences. The mentor-learner relationship is dynamic and complex, and effective learning occurs when this relationship is built on guided participation. This involves the mentor actively engaging with the learner, offering feedback, and facilitating the learner's growth and development within the professional practice.

Educational Content

The following topics are covered during the didactic section of an educational course on CVADs:

1. Anatomy and physiology of relevant body systems involved during CVADs
2. Ultrasound for initial assessment of the central veins to be used for the cannulation and for the insertion of the CVAD
3. Central venous device tip location and navigation by ultrasound (transthoracic echo) or by intracavitary electrocardiogram
4. Infection control and sterile technique
5. Device selection and indications
6. Mechanical complication prevention, evaluation, and management
7. Post-insertion care and maintenance practices of CVADs
8. Simulation training (inanimate models and virtual reality)

The recommended structure of an educational course on central venous catheterisation should include 6–8 h of didactic education, 4 h of hands-on training on inanimate models, and 6 h of hands-on training on normal human volunteers to detect normal ultrasound anatomy. This training should be followed by supervised ultrasound cannulations and coaching the trainee during the procedure to achieve the required minimal skill competence with the lowest rate of complications.

Competence and Certification

Competence refers to possessing the necessary knowledge, skills, and judgment required to effectively perform a specific task. Competence in CVAD placement and maintenance should include completing a written test assessing the practitioner's cognitive level of the procedure. This written exam should be in conjunction with a visual exam to test the knowledge of normal versus abnormal vessels and a skills test using simulation to test the practitioner's ability to perform the procedure satisfactorily. The practitioner would then undertake observed procedures under the direct supervision of an experienced practitioner. Global rating scales and checklists are the two main approaches to rating technical performance.

Certification is when a regulatory body formally recognises an individual's competence in a specific area. It involves an assessment or examination to demonstrate proficiency, and it often requires ongoing education or training to maintain the certification.

Pearls and Highlights

The introduction of ultrasound guidance in central venous cannulation has improved safety, but it is not the only solution to improve the outcome of this procedure.

- Magnetic guidance and photoacoustic needles can enhance the precision of needle tip visualisation, avoiding posterior wall puncture and reducing the time to cannulation.
- The use of assisted reality combined with ultrasound images allows better hand-eye coordination and focusing on the manoeuvre, directing the needle trajectory to the target vessel.
- Guidelines for CLABSI prevention have been created, but they have not yet been fully implemented in clinical practice. Education of healthcare providers is the key to reducing this complication.
- Education on central venous catheterisation has to be structured with objective goals that trainees must achieve before being considered competent and certified by board societies.

References

1. Boulet N, et al. How to improve the efficiency and the safety of real-time ultrasound-guided central venous catheterization in 2023: a narrative review. Ann Intensive Care. 2023;13(1):46.
2. Nakazawa H, et al. Use of a photoacoustic needle improves needle tip recognition in a video recording of simulated ultrasound-guided vascular access: a pilot study. J Vasc Access. 2024;25(3):922–7.
3. Arya V, et al. Comparative evaluation of success of ultrasound-guided internal jugular vein cannulation using needle with guard: a randomized, controlled study. J Anaesthesiol Clin Pharmacol. 2020;36(1):57–61.
4. Wu TS, Dameff CJ, Tully JL. Ultrasound-guided central venous access using Google Glass. J Emerg Med. 2014;47(6):668–75.
5. Lim H, et al. Use of smart glasses for ultrasound-guided peripheral venous access: a randomized controlled pilot study. Clin Exp Emerg Med. 2019;6(4):356–61.
6. Nguyen T, et al. HoloUS: augmented reality visualization of live ultrasound images using HoloLens for ultrasound-guided procedures. Int J Comput Assist Radiol Surg. 2022;17(2):385–91.
7. Panidapu N, et al. Internal jugular vein cannulation using a 3-dimensional ultrasound probe in patients undergoing cardiac surgery: comparison between biplane view and short-axis view. J Cardiothorac Vasc Anesth. 2021;35(1):91–7.
8. Jones NA, et al. Impact of a novel biplane user interface on ultrasound-guided vascular access performance: a prospective, randomized, crossover study. Med J (Ft Sam Houst Tex). 2023;(Per 23–4/5/6):25–30.
9. Scholten HJ, et al. 3D biplane versus conventional 2D ultrasound imaging for internal jugular vein cannulation. Intensive Care Med. 2022;48(2):236–7.
10. Walser EM. Venous access ports: indications, implantation technique, follow-up, and complications. Cardiovasc Intervent Radiol. 2012;35(4):751–64.
11. Lennon M, et al. Procedural complications of central venous catheter insertion. Minerva Anestesiol. 2012;78(11):1234–40.
12. Eisen LA, et al. Mechanical complications of central venous catheters. J Intensive Care Med. 2006;21(1):40–6.

13. Allegranzi B, et al. Burden of endemic health-care-associated infection in developing countries: systematic review and meta-analysis. Lancet. 2011;377(9761):228–41.
14. Rosenthal VD, et al. International Nosocomial Infection Control Consortium (INICC) report of health care associated infections, data summary of 45 countries for 2015 to 2020, adult and pediatric units, device-associated module. Am J Infect Control. 2024;52:1002.
15. Centers for Disease Control and Prevention. Vital signs: central line-associated blood stream infections--United States, 2001, 2008, and 2009. MMWR Morb Mortal Wkly Rep. 2011;60(8):243–8.
16. Rosenthal VD, et al. Multinational prospective study of incidence and risk factors for central-line-associated bloodstream infections in 728 intensive care units of 41 Asian, African, Eastern European, Latin American, and Middle Eastern countries over 24 years. Infect Control Hosp Epidemiol. 2023:1–11. https://doi.org/10.1017/ice.2023.69.
17. Rosenthal V, Memish Z, Shweta F, Bearman G, Lutwick L. Recommendations for the prevention of central line-associated bloodstream infections. In: Guide to infection control in the healthcare setting. Boston: International Society for Infectious Diseases; 2024.
18. Buetti N, et al. Strategies to prevent central line-associated bloodstream infections in acute-care hospitals: 2022 update. Infect Control Hosp Epidemiol. 2022;43(5):553–69.
19. Chopra V, et al. The Michigan Appropriateness Guide for Intravenous Catheters (MAGIC): results from a multispecialty panel using the RAND/UCLA appropriateness method. Ann Intern Med. 2015;163(6_Supplement):S1–S40.
20. Fakih MG, et al. First step to reducing infection risk as a system: evaluation of infection prevention processes for 71 hospitals. Am J Infect Control. 2013;41(11):950–4.
21. Owings A, et al. Leadership line care rounds: application of the engage, educate, execute, and evaluate improvement model for the prevention of central line-associated bloodstream infections in children with cancer. Am J Infect Control. 2018;46(2):229–31.
22. Pronovost PJ, Berenholtz SM, Needham DM. Translating evidence into practice: a model for large scale knowledge translation. BMJ. 2008;337:a1714.
23. Moureau N, et al. Evidence-based consensus on the insertion of central venous access devices: definition of minimal requirements for training. Br J Anaesth. 2013;110(3):347–56.
24. Lamperti M, et al. European Society of Anaesthesiology guidelines on peri-operative use of ultrasound-guided for vascular access (PERSEUS vascular access). Eur J Anaesthesiol. 2020;37(5):344–76.
25. Peltan ID, et al. Simulation improves procedural protocol adherence during central venous catheter placement: a randomized controlled trial. Simul Healthc. 2015;10(5):270–6.
26. Hameeteman M, et al. Ultrasound-guided central venous catheter placement by surgical trainees: a safe procedure? J Vasc Access. 2010;11(4):288–92.
27. Okano H, et al. Outcomes of simulation-based education for vascular access: a systematic review and meta-analysis. Cureus. 2021;13(8):e17188.
28. Latif RK, et al. Teaching aseptic technique for central venous access under ultrasound guidance: a randomized trial comparing didactic training alone to didactic plus simulation-based training. Anesth Analg. 2012;114(3):626–33.
29. Varga S, et al. Central venous catheterization using a perfused human cadaveric model: application to surgical education. J Surg Educ. 2015;72(1):28–32.
30. Jang Y-E, et al. Smart glasses for radial arterial catheterization in pediatric patients: a randomized clinical trial. Anesthesiology. 2021;135(4):612–20. https://doi.org/10.1097/ALN.0000000000003914.

MIX
Papier aus verantwortungsvollen Quellen
Paper from responsible sources
FSC® C105338

If you have any concerns about our products,
you can contact us on
ProductSafety@springernature.com

In case Publisher is established outside the EU,
the EU authorized representative is:
Springer Nature Customer Service Center GmbH
Europaplatz 3, 69115 Heidelberg, Germany

Printed by Libri Plureos GmbH
in Hamburg, Germany